The Complexities of Care

A VOLUME IN THE SERIES

The Culture and Politics of Health Care Work

Edited by Suzanne Gordon and Sioban Nelson

From Silence to Voice: What Nurses Know and Must Communicate to the Public,
  Second Edition
By Bernice Buresh and Suzanne Gordon

Nobody's Home: Candid Reflections of a Nursing Home Aide
By Thomas Edward Gass

Nursing against the Odds: How Health Care Cost Cutting, Media Stereotypes, and
  Medical Hubris Undermine Nurses and Patient Care
By Suzanne Gordon

Nurses on the Move: Migration and the Global Health Care Economy
By Mireille Kingma

Code Green: Money-Driven Hospitals and the Dismantling of Nursing
By Dana Beth Weinberg

The Complexities of Care

NURSING RECONSIDERED

EDITED BY

Sioban Nelson

and **Suzanne Gordon**

ILR Press
AN IMPRINT OF
CORNELL UNIVERSITY PRESS
ITHACA AND LONDON

An early version of chapter one appeared in the *American Journal of Nursing* 105, no. 5 (May 2005): 62–69, and is adapted here with permission.

First published 2006 by Cornell University Press
First printing, Cornell Paperbacks, 2006

Printed in the United States of America

Library of Congress Cataloging-in-Publication Data

The complexities of care : nursing reconsidered / edited by Sioban
    Nelson and Suzanne Gordon.
      p. cm. — (The culture and politics of health care work)
    Includes bibliographical references and index.
    ISBN-13: 978-0-8014-4505-7 (cloth : alk. paper)
    ISBN-10: 0-8014-4505-1 (cloth : alk. paper)
    ISBN-13: 978-0-8014-7322-7 (pbk. : alk. paper)
    ISBN-10: 0-8014-7322-5 (pbk. : alk. paper)
    1. Nursing. 2. Nursing—Philosophy. 3. Nursing ethics. 4. Nursing
—Social aspects. 5. Care of the sick. I. Nelson, Sioban.
II. Gordon, Suzanne, 1945– . III. Series.
    [DNLM: 1. Nursing Care. 2. Philosophy, Nursing. 3. Ethics,
Nursing. WY 100 C7375 2006]
RT82.C655 2006
610.73—dc22   2006006528

Cloth printing   10 9 8 7 6 5 4 3 2 1

Paperback printing   10 9 8 7 6 5 4 3 2 1

For Fran

Contents

Acknowledgments   ix

Introduction
Sioban Nelson and Suzanne Gordon   1

1. Moving beyond the Virtue Script in Nursing: Creating a
   Knowledge-Based Identity for Nurses   13
   Suzanne Gordon and Sioban Nelson

2. When Little Things Are Big Things: The Importance of
   Relationships for Nurses' Professional Practice   30
   Dana Beth Weinberg

3. Pride and Prejudice: Nurses' Struggle with Reasoned Debate   44
   Diana J. Mason

4. Moral Integrity and Regret in Nursing   50
   Lydia L. Moland

5. Ethical Expertise and the Problem of the Good Nurse   69
   Sioban Nelson

6. From Sickness to Health   88
   Tom Keighley

7. The New Cartesianism: Dividing Mind and Body and
   Thus Disembodying Care   *104*
   Suzanne Gordon

8. Nurses Must Be Clever to Care
   Sanchia Aranda and Rosie Brown   *122*

9. "You Don't Want to Stay Here": Surgical Nursing and the
   Disappearance of Patient Recovery Time   *143*
   Marie Heartfield

10. Research on Nurse Staffing and Its Outcomes: The Challenges
    and Risks of Grasping at Shadows   *161*
    Sean Clarke

    Conclusion: Nurses Wanted: Sentimental Men and Women Need
    Not Apply   *185*
    Sioban Nelson and Suzanne Gordon

    Notes   *191*
    Contributors   *203*
    Index   *205*

Acknowledgments

This book owes a debt to the plenitude of conversations, debates, and arguments we have enjoyed with nurses, other health professionals, social scientists, and health care watchers, many of whom would have no idea as to the impact of these conversations on the development of our ideas and of this volume. Our heartfelt thanks are due to you all for your willingness to engage with these ideas and challenge our assumptions.

A few individuals who have been directly involved in the production of this text warrant specific mention. Rick Ferri (Maine), Mary Ellen Purkis (Victoria, Canada), and Michael McGillion (Toronto), were all involved in early iterations of this volume, and Mike generously provided feedback on the draft manuscript. Margaret Sandelowski of University of North Carolina, Chapel Hill, and Mary Chiarella of University Technology, Sydney, Australia, reviewed the manuscript for Cornell, and we are grateful for their insights and advice. Thanks go to Debbie Fleming of the University of Melbourne, who oversaw the organization of the volume with characteristic efficiency and tolerance. We would also like to thank Ange Romeo-Hall for her editorial input, along with the rest of the wonderful team at Cornell University Press for their energy and professionalism.

The Complexities of Care

Introduction

Sioban Nelson and Suzanne Gordon

Like all good projects *The Complexities of Care* began as a conversation. It was a conversation held by the editors of this book over several years, over many hours of long-distance calls, by e-mail and, of course, in person—across many cities of North America, Europe, Australia, and Asia. This conversation was a kind of mutual compulsion. It bound us in concern for what we saw happening to patient care, nursing work, nursing education, and the nursing profession, as well as about what we heard and read nursing say about itself.

Nursing, everyone believes, is *the* caring profession. Tomes of texts on caring line the walls of nursing schools and student shelves. Indeed, the discipline of nursing is often known as the "caring science." Because of their caring reputation, nurses top the polls as the most trustworthy professionals. Yet, in spite of what seems to be an endless outpouring of public support, in almost every country in the world nursing is under threat, in the practice setting and in the academic sector. Indeed, its standing as a regulated profession is constantly challenged.

In the practice setting, how nurses deliver care is under attack. In the United States, nurses are constantly fending off efforts to replace registered nurses with poorly educated workers. Nurses are under pressure to justify their very existence at the bedside. Nurses are floated from units in which they have great expertise to units in which they have little, because administrators seem not to grasp that a nurse is not simply an extra pair of hands and feet but also a knowledgeable worker with specific skills. This pattern is true all over the world as health care consultants try to sell administrators

new schemes that base cost-cutting and so-called efficiencies on the elimination of nurses at all levels of the organization. Sometimes efforts to cut
nursing care are so extreme that, were they not so serious, they would bor-
der on farce. For example, in Switzerland, the minister of Public Health for
the canton of Zurich has suggested that one way to cut costs would be to
have nurses turn their hospitalized patients less frequently. Apparently the
minister is unaware of how much it costs to heal a bedsore or what it takes
to prevent one.

In the academic setting, nursing is under threat because governments
and academic administrators are trying to deal with current and anticipated nursing shortages by widening the portals of entry into the profession. In North America, people can become advanced practice nurses without ever having practiced as a nurse. This model of advanced practice is
clearly not premised on the previous mastery of practice per se. There are
those, too, who are trying to make money on nursing—and supposedly
solve the nursing shortage—by creating new opportunities for lower-level
entrants into health care and nursing. In Australia, for example, nurses are
strongly resisting a government push to further deskill nursing work by
transforming the educational sector. Politicians have even suggested that
high school students be given credit for subjects undertaken during their
secondary education if they want to enter nursing programs. Moves are
also afoot to allow vocational students from any type of program to receive
nursing program credit for certain classes. They have suggested that someone studying to be a beautician would have acquired competencies in, for
instance, communication or infection control, which are now accepted for
credit in the nursing program—as if talking to a person about coloring her
hair is equal to talking to a cancer patient who is losing hers! By equating
hairdressing and nursing, they show a profound lack of understanding and
recognition of the complexity and specificity of the knowledge that is acquired in nursing school. Similar threats to the integrity of nursing programs exist in the United Kingdom and New Zealand.

Nursing has been at a disadvantage in the academy because of its relatively new position as a research discipline. New public university funding
frameworks in place in New Zealand, Hong Kong, the United Kingdom,
and Ireland and under discussion in Australia, Brazil, and a number of
other countries threaten to exacerbate this disadvantage. By linking university funding with set criteria on research performance that emphasize impact factors and citations—measures heavily biased toward the well-
established sciences—nursing, along with other applied disciplines such as
education and other clinical disciplines, rank as "weak." This rating, in

turn, affects the capacity of nurse researchers to attract funding, further diminishing the discipline's ranking as a research science.

The regulatory autonomy of nurses is jeopardized by the proliferation of generic workers, health workers, care assistants, and a variety of other newer, cheaper, unregulated, nonunionized workers. How can nursing be regulated when so many unregulated workers are now considered "nursing" personnel? Moreover, how will these workers be able to fight for better patient care if they do not have the collective power or legitimacy to challenge their working conditions, their wages, and their educational preparation or to credibly draw attention to patient care and safety issues? As nurses have learned through centuries of struggle, to mount such successful challenges requires a public understanding of the importance of nursing work and the possession of a credible voice and political networks. Unregulated workers have none of these things.

When we consider the public's relationship to nursing, an unrecognized paradox quickly emerges. The public says it trusts nurses, yet it seems to tolerate a relentless series of assaults on the integrity of the profession.

In our view, this paradox is neither accidental nor natural but, in great part, the logical consequence of the fact that nurses and their organizations place such a heavy emphasis on nursing's and nurses' virtues rather than on their knowledge and concrete contributions. Nursing today stresses the emotional and ethical aspects of its work and increasingly defines "caring" in very particular ways.

As we have talked over the years, we have become increasingly intrigued by the problems that this emphasis on caring can create for a profession that seems to be in an almost permanent state of crisis; that is constantly seeking public legitimacy, that longs to be an equal partner with medicine, and that has, over the past decade, suffered serious attacks led by hospital cost-cutters, health care policymakers, and politicians.

We've initiated this discussion of the complexities of care because we believe there are unintended consequences arising from the way nurses think about, talk about, and structure their work. The goal of this book is to explore the interaction between caring discourse, nursing practice, and the economic and political environment in which nurses practice today. One of the recurring themes of this collection of essays is the manner in which rhetoric shapes the way people view nurses and nursing practice. Because we take caring seriously we are concerned that discussions of nursing care tend to sentimentalize and decomplexify the skill and knowledge involved in nurses' interpersonal or relational work with patients. We therefore worry that caring discourse may leave nurses and nursing with no line of defense against the fiscal and economic rationalizers who threaten their daily practice.

This problem not only affects nurses' ability to get the financial resources to support good practice but it leaves them vulnerable to self-blame and guilt as economic rationalizers erode the environment in which nurses practice. Nurses have less and less time to do basic and urgent patient care, and even less time for intensive emotional work. Many nurses tell us they blame themselves for their inability to care. This is because many have been taught that caring is the "art of self" and exists within the individual nurse, disconnected from the concrete realities that shape nursing practice. If nursing is indeed the art of self it is not surprising that nurses blame themselves for institutional and social failings. Similarly we are concerned that a sentimentalized caring rhetoric also leads those patients and families who experience the results of cuts in nursing care to blame individual nurses rather than the system. Of course all professionals are responsible for their practice, but over the past decade or more economic changes in health care have overwhelmed nurses' ability to compensate for declining resources.

The focus on interpersonal relationships and emotional connection and educational activities also tends to overlook and devalue the hard work of physical care that nurses have traditionally given to their patients. In fact, some elaborations of caring discourse seem to place such an emphasis on the psychosocial and educational activities of the nurse that they entirely ignore the skills and complexity of body work. In the context of health service and workforce restructuring that constantly tries to replace higher skilled—and thus more expensive workers—with those who are less skilled and cheaper, this focus may enable administrators to justify farming out "softer" activities to unskilled workers and family members. All of which places patients at significant risk.

This book is made up of a series of essays that explore the challenges nurses face and how they respond to them. We consider the way nursing engages with these challenges at the philosophical level as well as how working nurses confront contemporary realities in their daily practice or in conversations with politicians, health care policymakers, journalists, and the public.

These essays raise a number of questions and explore a number of issues that have great relevance to the future of the profession and the practice of nursing. We are concerned that caring discourse, as it is currently constructed, may actually fragment the nursing workforce and undermine the ability of nurses to cohesively confront the problems they face. Over the years, for example, we have observed and known many excellent nurses who make significant contributions to patient care. In their daily practice, they don't, however, conform to the hand-holding images of emotional caring that the profession increasingly promotes. These are tough-minded women and men who talk about their technical and medical expertise and their pragmatic actions. But they are often dismissed as being somehow uncaring, not having the heart of a nurse, or being somehow inauthentic. As we have observed this trend, we have wondered how it is that caring has become so narrowly defined that using technology or medical knowledge to, for example, prevent complications of surgery or the disease process is not considered an act of caring.

When we listen to some nurses describe the rewards of their profession, many suggest that the primary reward a nurse gets is the "gratitude" she perceives in the eyes of the patient, or the human rewards of working with people for whom she feels "unconditional love." As one 2005 CD by Michael Stillwater and Gary Malkin, *Care for the Journey: Sustaining the Heart of Healthcare*, claims approvingly, people don't value nurses for their expertise but for their humanity (www.wisdomoftheworld.com/products). Listening to these dewy-eyed descriptions, we worry that the rewards available to nurses have drastically lessened. What happens to the nurse whose patient isn't grateful because he got her out of bed to walk after surgery? Or to the nurse who does a good technical job? Or the nurse who takes care of people whom she doesn't like? As one nurse recently put it, "I get so beaten down by all this talk about caring. I take care of some people I just can't stand. I don't care a hoot about them. I would prefer never to have seen them or never to see them again. What I care about is doing a really good job and giving really good physical care to all of my patients, including the ones I can't stand."

Indeed, we've noticed that some nurses seem to categorize their own colleagues according to how emotionally or sentimentally they behave—ranking those who seem to do more emotional work as being "real nurses" and downgrading those who do more technical work as not being "real nurses." Thus people who work in operating rooms (theater), emergency wards, in endoscopy, and even in intensive care units may be cast as the noncaring, not quite authentic nurses, while a nurse in oncology or psychiatry or community care becomes the prototypical caring, "real" nurse. What happens to the academic or nurse manager is even more interesting. She or he risks not being considered a nurse at all. Obviously, this emotional or sentimental ranking presents serious problems for a profession that is trying to maintain some sense of internal cohesion as it responds to threats on the fronts we have described.

What presents even more problems is how this self-description connects to what has happened in the health care workplace over the last few decades. We have learned from nurses around the world who are directly involved in the health care sector that all too often health care systems no longer support caring work. Even more disturbing, patients are experiencing nursing *care* that has little to justify its name. Many patients tell us—and some tell researchers—that the most "caring"—that is, emotionally attentive or kindly—people they come in contact with are not nurses at all but lower-level aides and hospital workers. Registered nurses, they tell us, don't seem to have time to talk, to be kind and gentle, to listen or express concern and compassion. So if RNs are supposed to be caring but have no time to care—to do emotional work—does that mean that they are not really authentic nurses? And if the nurses don't have time to do emotional work—and the rest of their work is invisible—have they failed? Are they no longer real nurses?

What we have also noticed and find of even greater concern is the opposite side of this sentimental coin—some nurses appear to value roles that remove them from the clinical field or from direct patient care. Have many nurses been seduced by the idea that the new powerful nurse is the coordinator or leader of care—*not* the caregiver? Care, whatever this is, has begun to sink from nursing's view and to have become the work of others.

In our discussions we elaborated many manifestations of this phenomenon and pondered its implications. What does it mean to be caring? What is the nurse-patient relationship all about? On what is it grounded? Should we be worried about it at all? Does it matter who delivers care? Are the realms of advanced practice such as clinical nurse leader roles, nurse practitioners, and doctorates of nursing practice in fact the future of the profession, and is the coordination of less skilled workers a sensible response to the human resource crisis that dominates nursing workforce issues in most of the world? Maybe so, but if so then why do we keep talking so much about care and what does any of it mean anymore?

One possible explanation that we explore in a number of chapters is that the holistic rhetoric that dominates so much of nursing discourse means that it is almost impossible for nurses to talk about their work in any other way.

We approach the questions and issues we raise from a number of perspectives and points of view. These are reflected in the choice of contributors who come from a variety of different countries and include nurses as well as others who are engaged with nursing and caregiving issues. One of the coeditors of this book is a journalist who has spent the past two decades observing and writing about nursing; one contributor is a sociologist who has studied the impact of cost-cutting and hospital mergers on the nursing workforce; another contributor is a philosopher who has written about moral integrity in professional work. The fact that nonnurses exhibit such a deep concern for the future of nursing and the rhetoric of nursing theory and practice underlines how important nursing is not only to nurses themselves but to those who depend on nursing care. Similarly, that nurses and observers in the United States, Australia, and Great Britain are all concerned about these issues shows that they defy neat national borders and are, with some cultural variations, common in much of the world.

Over the course of ten chapters the authors squarely address what we consider to be the major challenges confronting nurses engaged in practice. Several chapters deal directly with the disconnect between talking the talk and walking the walk when nurses talk and think about what they do and how they interact with their patients. Others look at the philosophical issues that confront the discipline of nursing and how these issues help or hinder nurses in their practice and in the development of a better health system.

In our first chapter the two editors of this book, a nurse and nonnurse, describe the power of what we call the "virtue script" in nursing. When asked to describe or justify their work, nurses all too often rely on traditional caring discourse that presents the nurse as the good, trusting, compassionate figure, failing to recognize the knowledge and skill that nurses must have in order to care for patients. We raise concerns that with its images of hearts, hands, and angels this virtue script sentimentalizes and trivialize what is in fact complex and highly skilled knowledge work.

As Patricia Benner has frequently pointed out, nurses' emotional work requires significant expertise. Our essay examines the complex process of professional self-definition that has become the language nurses mobilize when talking about their work and the importance of nursing care to patients and to the health care system. We explore the historical evolution of the nurse as virtue worker and the development of what we term the "feedback loop," through which this image has been reproduced and reinforced. After examining the virtue script in contemporary media representations of nursing and high-profile recruitment campaigns, such as the Johnson & Johnson Campaign for Nursing's Future, we conclude with concrete suggestions for a more effective and accurate recruitment message that reframes nursing as knowledge work that will not only attract new recruits but will retain them at the bedside or in other areas of direct patient care.

The way nursing discourse hampers nurses' attempts to protect the nurse-patient relationship and the integrity of nursing services in hospitals is the theme of U.S. sociologist Dana Weinberg's powerful essay on the dismantling of the nursing service at the Beth Israel Hospital in Boston. Weinberg elaborates on her ground-breaking book, *Code Green*, by highlighting and analyzing the way in which a narrowed caring discourse prevented nurses from defending one of the most successful models of nursing care delivery developed in the twentieth century. She argues that when nurses at Beth Israel confronted administrators determined to cut costs by slashing nursing, the nurses were unable to clearly articulate what they brought to patient care in a language that hospital administrators concerned only with the bottom line could understand.

Diana Mason continues this exploration as she considers how difficult it is to generate, within the profession, a more critical debate about the images and discourse nurses use to promote their work and claim their social legitimacy. As editor in chief of the *American Journal of Nursing*, Mason has tried to encourage a critical debate in its pages. This has been difficult, she believes, because nurses so often argue not about ideas but against the people who voice them. She bases her analysis on the causes of a heated response to several publications that ran in the *American Nursing Journal* in 2004. Readers reacted angrily to portrayals of nurses as less than pure and virtuous. Stifling rather than advancing the critical thinking nurses are encouraged to do today, readers attacked the author, the journal, and its editors. The message: Woe betide anyone who tries to present a more gritty or realistic image of nursing.

In the next essay we move to philosophical considerations. Adding another dimension to this discussion of how nurses present their work to a wider public, U.S. philosopher Lydia Moland brings attention to the moral dilemma nurses experience when they find that they are unable to reconcile the caring and holistic values of the profession with their daily work inside a pressured, uncaring, and unholistic health care system. Again, how they express the contradictions in their work and their sense of what Moland calls "moral integrity" determines how people outside of nursing view the profession.

Keeping this philosophical framing, Sioban Nelson's essay retains the focus on the tension between nursing practice and knowledge. What is the relationship between ethical practice and the ethical individual? Are good nurses ipso facto "good" people? Taking issue with a particular construct of ethical expertise as proposed by Patricia Benner and other thinkers Nelson challenges the idea that ethical and clinical expertise can be categorized along a novice-to-expert continuum. She raises concerns about the way in which ethical debates in nursing privilege the ideal of the expert nurse who always simply "knows" the right course of action, while ignoring the systemic issues that confound working nurses.

Tom Keighley's chapter argues that one of the real problems confronting nursing today is the overarching effect of "health" discourse. Keighley analyses the mission statements of many prominent national and international nursing organizations and finds that very few of them include the care of the sick as part of their mission. What they are after, he explains, is the pursuit of health. As health care systems around the world are under increasing pressure to reinvent themselves as efficient and economically sustainable, the discourses of health and of patient self-management provide the language to erase the health system's core mission of caring for the sick and vulnerable. What happens to patients, Keighley asks, when nursing is silent about the care of the sick, its traditional mandate? He argues that nursing's enthusiasm for this pursuit of health and its retreat from sickness arose as an unintended consequence of nursing's endorsement of the Declaration of Alma-Ata of 1978, which defined health as a human right and achievable goal. This shift in thinking also coincided with major restructuring of health care systems in the 1980s and 1990s that ended the Nightingale system of nurse-led and directed line management. Keighley explores the significant problems that nurses and their patients encounter when nursing's focus and major concern is health almost to the exclusion of sickness.

Through all of the changes in and challenges to nursing over the past three decades one idea has been a consistent and powerful theme—that of holism. Suzanne Gordon's essay on holism centers on a surprising paradox. She argues that an unintended consequence of nursing's focus on holism has been a loss of the ability or even the desire to present a truly holistic description of nursing practice. Instead, from academia to the practice setting nurses' discussion of their holistic practice obscures its breadth and complexity and conceals the range of medical, technical, and emotional skills and knowledge nurses possess. Suzanne Gordon argues that holistic discourse reproduces rather than overcomes the Cartesian divide between mind and body. She contends that holism represents a new Cartesianism in nursing that constructs a myth about the purpose and meaning of the nurse-patient relationship that may compromise nurses' attempts to effectively defend their practice.

It is the very question of nursing work that the next contributors, Sanchia Aranda and Rosie Brown, confront. In this essay we move into a practice setting dominated by cost-cutting and persistent attempts to deliver less expensive nursing care. Aranda and Brown report on field research in palliative care that shows a clinical and caring deskilling of nurses, who, under service restructuring directives, begin to view themselves as coordinators of care rather than caregivers. They raise central questions about how nurses themselves are being taught to view the nurse-patient relationship and its purpose. They argue that it is by talking to patients about their problems or while delivering hands-on care that nurses get to know, understand, and thus clinically assess their patients. Their fieldwork revealed a worrying trend. Nurses lose those assessment skills when their role is redefined from that of clinical hands-on caregiver to the care coordinator or case manager. They are concerned about this little-commented-on but critical erosion of "bedside" skill and argue compellingly for a strong foundation in basic nursing at all levels of practice—for nursing students, new graduates, and experienced nurses. Without mentors and role models how will tomorrow's nurses reach a level of comfort and confidence with intimate physical care that is essential for good patient management?

Australian nurse-researcher Marie Heartfield continues to explore the practice realm as she looks at the imperatives of health care cost-cutting from another vantage point. She considers the way in which nurses working on short-stay units are encouraged to view their patients and argues that as nursing work has been radically restructured nurses are now forced to (and sometimes embrace) what could be considered to be anticaring practices. This essay, which was drawn from a larger study the author conducted on the impact of economic rationalization in health care, examines the transformation that has taken place in the last decade in the way many nurses view patients and define their patients' needs. In her study she found that nurses were taught to redefine patients as sick enough to require surgery but somehow well enough to take care of themselves. She looks at the implications of caring discourse as it relates to the dilemmas these nurses faced. Although the focus on caring can be mobilized to encourage nurses to fight for the full range of services and attention that patients need, it can also be used as a smokescreen that prevents nurses from confronting the implications of service restructuring for the care they deliver. In fact, if nurses consider themselves to be unquestionably caring, they can fall into the trap of denying that at times nurses do some very uncaring things.

Sean Clarke concludes this collection with an important essay that raises critical questions about the way in which we understand nursing work. Clarke, who has worked with Linda Aiken at the University of Pennsylvania on landmark studies that connect nursing staffing levels and patient mortality, weighs in on one of the most vexing issues that arises when nurses contemplate solutions to the nursing crisis: the debate about staffing ratios or how many nurses it takes to keep patients safe. As he considers the role of the researcher, Clarke talks about the limitations researchers face in analyzing the nursing workforce and the effects of nursing activities on patient care. He warns us about making too much of the numbers as well as not enough of them. Easily overlooked in researchers' rush to fill the log of nursing activities, measure their importance, and justify the central place of a skilled and educated nursing workforce in a quality health care system are a number of vital epistemological and methodological questions. Clarke asks, "What do we know about nursing and how do we know it?" Taking us inside the research process, he points out how difficult it is to measure what nurses do and how they do it. As a result many researchers must be content with measuring only the traces of what we understand nursing work to be. Yet how we measure these traces in turn defines how we then understand nursing work. Clarke talks about how not enough researchers want to study—or can find the funds to study—the daily work of bedside nurses, and he sets out a series of challenges for future research in caregiving.

In our final chapter we argue that the cost of caring should not fall only on the shoulders of nurses but on society as a whole. In a society that values care of the sick, there will not be a shortage of nurses. The challenge for nursing as a profession is to ensure that it does not work against these ends by adding to the overwhelming burden individual nurses carry as a result of our respective health care systems' failure to provide sufficient resources for quality care. We urge the profession to embrace and own the scientific and technical ability of the skilled nurse; to communicate the importance of one of the health care system's best patient-safety device—the registered nurse; and to appreciate the critical value of all working nurses, whether in advanced practice or as a new nursing school graduate or as a member of the global workforce that cares for the sick and promotes health.

Throughout this volume we and the other authors critique the caring discourse that has become the currency of modern nursing. Lest we and some of our authors be accused to being anticaring, not understanding the importance of things that cannot be measured, not understanding nursing, or attacking the human project of giving emotional support to the sick and vulnerable, we want to clearly state our point of view. We believe that the kind of emotional and social support nurses provide patients is critical. We don't believe everything can be counted, described, or scientifically analyzed. But we do believe that caring discourse has been uncritically accepted as dogma rather than critically described or explored. In so much of the dogma, the historical roots and purposes of caring discourse are ignored, its contemporary impact discounted; and what caring brings patients is sometimes lost in a sea of saccharine. Most important—and we cannot say this strongly enough—much of the contemporary "virtue script" trivializes what are in fact complex skills. It makes the caring that nurses give appear to be feeling as opposed to cognitive work and thus it paves the way for nice—rather than educated—women, or men, to replace the educated, experienced nurses who, we believe, are critical to patient care.

As the editors, we're pleased to be able to present a range of critical perspectives on major issues in nursing and health care work. We believe that it's important for all those who work in nursing, who study nursing, and who are concerned about the future of health care to be prepared to have their views challenged and their thinking stimulated. We include ourselves and our contributors in this endeavor.

1

Moving beyond the Virtue Script in Nursing

Creating a Knowledge-Based Identity for Nurses

Suzanne Gordon and Sioban Nelson

Nursing is facing a major worldwide crisis. The nursing workforce is aging. The profession is plagued by poor rates of nurse retention in hospitals and other health care institutions. Because of changes in women's roles, it is more and more difficult to attract the traditional recruit–young women—to nursing. Nursing has also been stubbornly unable to change the proportion of men in the profession. A recent report in the journal *Health Affairs* found, for example, that young men are leaving the profession at twice the rate of their female counterparts.[1] These factors, combined with an aging population and soaring rates of chronic illness that demand active care and management, are producing a global nursing shortage of potentially devastating dimensions. The United States and Canada, to cite just two examples, will face a shortfall of one million and 113,000 nurses respectively in the next decade and a half.

This shortage has now galvanized nursing organizations, unions, health care policymakers, political representatives, foundations, corporations, and governments. There is, not surprisingly, a difference of opinion over the causes of and possible solutions to the current crisis. Unions argue that government regulations and contract language must mandate concrete changes in working conditions—through measures such as bans on mandatory overtime, implementation of mandatory nurse-to-patient staffing ratios, and increases in pay—if the shortage is to be remedied. Other groups believe that increasing the supply of nurses, producing more educated, so-called advanced practice nurses or nurse leaders, and providing health care institutions with financial incentives to create new models of nursing care delivery will solve the problem. No matter where they stand along this spectrum of solutions, most nurses agree that any action to support nursing and increase recruitment to the profession depends, in part, on a better public understanding of nurses' scientific knowledge and clinical skill and thus their centrality to patient care—a connection made in a number of recent scientific studies published in prestigious medical and nursing journals.[2]

To present a more modern image of nursing and publicize their solutions to the nursing crisis, dozens of groups have produced advertising campaigns and promotional messages designed to attract new recruits to the profession. An analysis of the messages in this promotional material reveals, however, that claims for clinical significance of nursing knowledge and skill are constantly undercut by the reliance on messages that stress nursing's *moral* legitimacy and nurses' virtuous behavior. Although an increasing number of studies by nursing, medical, and public health researchers have documented the link between nursing care and lower rates of hospital-acquired infections, falls, bedsores, deep-vein thrombosis, pulmonary emboli and deaths, most promotional campaigns are conspicuous for their failure to integrate this data into their messages. Instead, they tend to reinforce nursing's "old image" as good work performed by kind and nice people (women), as opposed to skilled and intelligent work. It is this juxtaposition between heart and head, between virtue versus knowledge work, that is the subject of this chapter.

Nursing image has, of course, been much studied over the past decades. Research has shown that nurses are consistently left out of media reports on health care and tend to be covered only when there is a strike or shortage.[3] What is rarely addressed in discussions of nursing image is how nurses themselves reinforce traditional images of their work. Similarly the historical origins and reasons for their choice of verbal and visual images have been poorly explored.

The question that we address here, thus, moves beyond a critique of the media and professional portraiture of nurses and nursing work to examine the historical formation of the image of nursing as virtue work and the abiding appeal and power of this image over nursing and nurses.

To understand this dynamic we examine the historical formation of nursing as a virtuous practice and discuss how this focus on virtue helped nurses overcome a number of nineteenth-century obstacles to the advancement of women and the professionalization of nursing. We then discuss the constitution of nursing as virtue work in the contemporary representation and framing of nursing practice. Finally, we argue that, in the contemporary context, when nurses are under tremendous pressure to justify their practice in terms of outcomes and efficiencies, the virtue script prevents nursing from gaining the respect it has long sought. It also hinders the effort to recruit and retain new candidates who will not only enter but will remain in the profession over the long term. Indeed, this virtue script sets up a powerful feedback loop through which nurses project archaic images to the public. The public, media, and other professionals, and even patients in their turn, reflect this image of nursing as virtue work back to nurses. This social process produces the lens through which nursing is still seen and understood.

Power of Angels—Past

Modern nursing emerged in the nineteenth century in part because urbanization and industrialization created a surfeit of women who needed or wanted to work outside the home. The increasing distress of the poor associated with this urbanization and industrialization also led to the rise of philanthropic movements of single, educated women whose religious fervor and passion for reform led them to enter the world as independent social actors. Finally, nursing was deeply influenced by the development of scientific medicine and, its corollary, the modern hospital.[4]

From the contemporary vantage point, it is difficult to recapture the extent to which the idea of a female profession was a radical proposition in the nineteenth century. For most women marriage—which merely transferred a woman's bondage to her husband —was the only release from a father's authority. Moving beyond the patriarchal home to perform a role in the public world was, for respectable women, only possible in prescribed ways. Catholic women were able to enter a convent if they had the suitable background and education plus the required dowry. A few respectable women who needed to work outside of the home could get jobs as governesses, which to a great extent turned them into servants of well-to-do families. Women who wanted to work as nurses thus confronted novel problems in social relations and decorum. The pressing problem for them was dealing with men, all men—patients, medical students, surgeons and physicians, hospitals managers, and boards of governors.

Nurses were paid to work with the sick bodies of strangers mostly male strangers, who were the majority of patients in nineteenth-century hospitals.[5] To do their work, nurses gained knowledge of anatomical processes (reproduction, elimination, and so forth). In an era that prized "blushing innocence" as a feminine virtue, this kind of knowledge was considered inappropriate for women. Whether on the battlefields, in hospitals, or in the homes of both rich and poor, nurses were confronted with unpleasant, unladylike realities—such as poverty and disease. This experience threatened their respectability by subjecting them to the stigma of moral and physical contamination.

To confront the obstacles they faced in negotiating professional and male-female social relationships, nurse reformers followed the pathway opened for them by religious nurses. Protected and desexualized by veil and vow, a large number of women followed religious vocations in Catholic and Protestant Europe and North America in the early nineteenth century. In order to navigate new areas of gendered social relations, secular nurses too relied on this template. To desexualize and make the nurse respectable, they modified veils and cornettes into the nurse's cap, and nuns' habits into the drab, starched uniform of the Nightingale nurse. They retained the custom of using the title "sister" to denote a respectable, educated nurse, and—perhaps most importantly—they emphasized nursing as essentially a calling or vocation in which virtue was its own reward. Nursing students were housed in cloisterlike dormitories and expected to remain single.

The religious counterparts of secular nurses were enjoined to "say little, do much," to exhibit personal and intellectual modesty, and to conceal their agency. They were not allowed to "own" anything, including their own knowledge. For instance, in 1889 Mother Superior Saint Pierre of San Antonio advised her nuns (who were working as teachers and nurses) to "remain hidden, Alphonse. I cannot recommend this as much as I would like to, and beg you to give this spirit to our sisters. It is better that people take us for imbeciles, in no matter what, than to consider us clever and intelligent, agreeable to popular or worldly opinion."[6] Well into the twentieth century secular nursing was also commonly depicted in such terms. Thus a nursing superintendent commented that "[nursing has] opened up . . . rich opportunities of service to others, while in the world, not a part of it . . . because she [the nursing student] is shielded and her associates are those engaged in the same unselfish work."[7]

Constituting nursing as altruistic, charitable, and self-sacrificing work—work that was "in but not of the world"—was fundamental to both removing its social stigma and desexualizing the individual nurse. It was this that allowed thousands of women to immerse themselves in the gritty realities of birth, life, and death and to work with bodies. This almost religious purpose elevated both nurses' work and the nurse who did it above the stigma of hard work, infection risk, and contaminated bodies. It also allowed nursing to become the first social activity of women outside the home that succeeded in gaining acceptance among the respectable classes and that ultimately helped women move into other professions.[8] Equally important, the constitution of nursing as virtue as opposed to knowledge work furnished secular nurses with an important arm in their battle with medicine and male doctors over what was to become, by the late nineteenth century, the highly contested terrain of the modern hospital.

Contested Space

In the first part of the nineteenth century medicine little resembled the monolith of scientific and professional power that it had become by the twentieth. In fact, early in the century the patent failure of medicine to assist during times of great calamity—such as during cholera outbreaks—lead to great criticism of physicians.[9] All of that changed with breakthroughs in science, anesthetics, and surgery. The medical profession galvanized around scientific practice, excluding empirics, homeopaths, midwives, and other "irregular practitioners," and rapid advances were made in its consolidation and development.[10]

Medicine, which was just gaining social legitimacy, was threatened by movements for female emancipation and education. These movements included not only women who wanted to be doctors but nurses who wanted more training, education, and authority. Many physicians were not welcoming to newly confident nurse reformers who were trying to improve the hospital and professionalize its nursing staff. From Britain to the United States to Australia, the story of hospital and nursing reform is thus characterized by political battles between medical and nursing leaders and by the medical and business allies of both groups.

One of the famous battles was between prominent English doctors and Florence Nightingale and her peers who proposed a model that gave nurses professional independence in the sphere of nursing and hospital management. Doctors and their political supporters insisted that nurses were no more than physicians' servants. In a letter to The Times, physicians presented one of the most unequivocal expressions of medicine's view of nurses:

> The medical argument is . . . that nursing is merely one of the means of cure, like the administration of medicines or the performance of operations; and that, like these, it can only be rightly carried out under absolute and unconditional subjection, in every principle and detail, to the doctor who is responsible for the case.[11]

A nurse's proper role was to follow doctors' orders in everything from applying a poultice to "the placing of a pillow."[12] She was to be a "passive agent," to give doctors "that cordial submissive cooperation which complete sympathy alone can insure."[13] She was also to embody the kind of self-sacrificing, devotion that, according to the bishop of Rochester, made of the hospital not only a "place of pain" but a "place of joy . . . where there were angels in human form earning happiness and giving happiness."[14] These attitudes toward nursing are far from quaint and dated, as we will soon see.

Nursing—A Moral Action

Faced with medical opposition and patriarchal assumptions, nursing reformers used the means and arguments at their disposal and mobilized the Victorian view that women possessed a superior moral power and essential female virtues that could be mobilized for the commonweal.

In the mid-nineteenth century, before the establishment of germ theory, Florence Nightingale built her campaign for the reform of nursing on two pillars. As a follower of the famed public health reformer, Edwin Chadwick, Nightingale believed that the cause of sickness and death was the filth and disorder that produced "miasma," through a yeast-like process that poisoned the air and corrupted the bodies of those with whom it came into contact. Cleanliness and order were thus the principal remedies for the widespread social and physical ills of the mid-nineteenth century.[15] Nightingale married these sanitarian concerns to the Victorian ideal of a separate sphere and moral role for women in the hospital. Influenced by successful religious nurses and their hospitals, Nightingale wanted the secular hospital to be managed by a matron or lady superintendent, replacing the husband and wife team of master and mistress who had generally managed hospitals from the time of the Reformation.[16]

Trained and educated nurses, however, were not the only contenders to replace the master and mistress of the old hospitals. The medicalization of hospitals from philanthropic to clinical institutions that took place over the last decades of the nineteenth century brought with it calls for medical direction and authority. Debate ensued as to whether nurses should report to the lady superintendent or to physicians. The level of authority of the lady superintendent was also subject to much debate.[17] Proponents of scientific medicine insisted that nurses should answer to physicians and were convinced of the "right" of a medical men to run the hospital. To counter medical opposition, Nightingale and her sister reformers used, as historian Charles Rosenberg has described it, "a powerful, well-calculated appeal for public and medical support."[18] They promoted the reforming power of the good nurse, who would bring order, efficiency, and the appropriate moral tone to the chaos of the nineteenth-century hospital—and who would, by the twentieth century, as students, provide the hospital with a cheap source of labor.[19]

Reformers in Britain, the United States, Australia, Canada, and France all stressed the moral, feminine virtues of the nurse. Prior to World War I, French nursing reformers assured doctors and government bureaucrats that the secular nurses who replaced religious nurses would have the appropriate "feminine tenderness of spirit" and that they would "furnish personnel with the same guarantees (as religious orders) of aptitude and devotion."[20] In the United States, nurse reformers such as Isabel Hampton Robb at Johns Hopkins Hospital defined nurses as "a physician's hand lengthened out to minister to the sick" and stressed the "nurturing function" of the nurse and "the highest belief in the mission of women as the superior moral force, and in the possibility of universal happiness."[21]

By the twentieth century the nurse had become defined by her:

> self-sacrifice, . . . devotion to duty, . . . all the domestic virtues. . . . Our young nurses must be inspired also with a keen sense of citizenship, so that when they leave training school they will be fully alive to the importance of their public and professional duties and ready to enter corporate life in the right spirit, the spirit which asks not what it is to receive but what it can give.[22]

Nursing clearly constituted itself as a feminine domain of moral authority and womanly skill. As the historian Charles Rosenberg has written, rather than arguing from a set of "discipline specific cognitive skills," nurses instead relied on "sacrifice, devotion and sensitivity, not intellect and decisiveness."[23] Thus, in order to create nursing as a profession that would be respectable enough to attract middle-class women who would not be a threat to medical authority, what took place was the downplaying of nursing knowledge and skill and the emphasizing of virtue and ethics. This meant that the very success of nurse reformers in creating the first mass profession for women put nurses in the paradoxical position of playing an important role in health care while sentimentalizing and trivializing the very critical role they played. The only legitimacy nurses could claim was by couching their description of their work in charitable, devotional, or altruistic terms.[24]

Virtue 1: The Power of Angels—Present

Women negotiating the path to professional pursuits and public respect arguably had few other scripts than that of virtue to follow in the late nineteenth and early twentieth centuries. What is, remarkable, however, is that this reliance on a virtue script has changed so little in the late twentieth and early twenty-first centuries as women have gained greater social, economic, legal, and political power. A sampling of campaigns—advertisements, videos, brochures, articles, newsletters, T-shirts, all of which not only describe but define nursing to the public—suggests that nurses are still grounding their claims for social legitimacy and respect on their virtues rather than their knowledge.

Consider the following excerpt from *Nursing: The Ultimate Adventure*, a video produced by the National Student Nurses Association for junior and senior high school students about the exciting career of registered professional nursing. While the video does make vague references to learning a lot and knowing a lot, what nurses learn and know is never specified. What is discussed at some length is how much public warmth and love they receive. Thus, Beverly Malone, at that time president of the American Nurses Association, declares: "The public loves me as a nurse and they don't even know my name but if I say I'm an RN, there's affection and warmth and an experience that means so much to me." She is then followed by a young woman who advises that "if you really want a job where people will love you," you should choose nursing.[25]

In 2002, to celebrate National Nurses Week, Ohio Health Systems produced a brochure with a gauzy picture of nurses wheeling a sick patient. The copy read:

> People believe there are beings
> That come to you in your darkest hour
> Guide you when your life hangs in the balance.
> Cradle you.
> Calm you.
> Protect you.
> Some people call them guardian angels.
> We call them nurses.[26]

In October 2001, *Nursing Profile*, a Michigan nursing magazine, ran an article on the accomplishments of an African American nurse, Birthale Archie, who has a master's degree in nursing. Rather than alerting the reader to the fact that this nurse was "educated to help others," the headline on the cover proclaimed "Born to Help Others—Black nurses' advocate Birthale Archie has volunteered her time and talent since childhood."[27]

The jingle for a televised public service announcement for the Nurses for a Healthier Tomorrow campaign, led by Sigma Theta Tau International (the nursing honor society), reads:

> What'll I do? What'll I be? Will I be the one who's there? Will I be providing care? Is it me who'll make the difference? Whatever I'll be, it'll be me. Building a better world. I'm building a better world. Nursing, it's Real. It's life.[28]

In 2000, the slogan for the Nurses Week campaign of the Quebec Order of Nurses was "Nursing—an expertise straight from the heart." In 2000, the Canadian Nurses Association's Nurses Week slogan was "Always there for you and your family." In 2002, the American Nurses Association (ANA) Nurses Week chose the tag line "Nurses Care for America" stamped across a heart bearing the stars and stripes, and in 2003, the ANA slogan was "Touching Lives, Lifting Spirits." The Federation of Nurses of Quebec (Federation des Infirmières et Infirmiers du Quebec) in 2003 played a new variation on this old theme, "Caring, the most noble work in the world." For Nurses Week 2002, the nursing school and hospital of the Medical University of South Carolina produced a brochure entitled "The Many Faces of Nursing." In it, are thirty-two short descriptions of their work written by nurses. The majority of these stories talk about nursing in terms its virtues. One nurse described "the little extra things you can do to make a difference . . . communicating with families, making them comfortable with pain meds or pillow fluffing." Another, which provided no details about the knowledge and clinical skills mobilized to care for a woman with HIV/AIDS did however stress that she and her patient had "become friends." Other stories talked about nurses who cried with patients and families. Interestingly, many highlighted nurses' sense of powerlessness. "I felt so helpless because there was so little I could do," one nurse commented. Nonetheless, she explained that "the family described me as an angel sent from God to help them get through this tragedy." Another talked not about the power of nursing skill and knowledge but the power of prayer.[29]

Even some of the feistiest, most assertive nursing campaigns rely on this virtue script. In 2001, the Massachusetts Nurses Association went on strike for safe staffing and better pay at the Brockton Hospital and won significant protections for nurses and patients. The T-shirt distributed to nurses and strike supporters proclaimed: "Nurses Make a Difference." To graphically depict that difference, the MNA chose to decorate these T-shirts with sunny, childlike pink, orange, blue, and green hearts.

These messages are so pervasive that they create a social feedback loop that reinforces and then reproduces the nineteenth-century view that nurses are sentimental workers who act as agents of a higher power (God or the doctor). Through this feedback loop nurses send virtue messages to other professionals, members of the public, patients, and the media. These groups, in their turn, broadcast these messages to an even wider public and then back to nursing.

In his introduction to the Nurses Week brochure cited above, the medical director of the Medical University of South Carolina described the role of nursing as follows:

We physicians at MUSC have much to appreciate in working with our nursing staff. Nurses amplify by their extended bedside presence the value of our brief daily patient encounters. The expertise and personal touch of our nurses drive much of the community's perception of our healthcare facilities. And the vigilance and judgment of our nurses permit us to travel to our daily duties and yet still respond to any sudden clinical event.[30]

Given the content of the stories included in the booklet, it would be difficult to counter this definition of nurses as agents of a higher power.

Faced with assertions from within nursing that it is "always there" or is an "expertise straight from the heart," it's not surprising that at the 2002 convention for Canadian nursing students, one of Canada's health care job fair companies presented nursing students with white T-shirts emblazoned with the logo, "I didn't know angels flew this low!"

Perhaps the most critical actor in this feedback loop is the mass media. When writing stories or headlines about nurses in newspapers and magazines, one sees nurses, when one sees them at all, as self-sacrificing, self-effacing angels of mercy. The *Toronto Star* produced a supplement for Nurses Week. The tabloid section included pictures of nurses at work. In one photo, a neonatal intensive care unit nurse sat surrounded by the high-tech paraphernalia of the ICU as she was rocking one of her tiny patients. The headline did not describe this highly skilled nurse as someone whose knowledge saves infants' lives every day. Instead, the caption introduced her as "St. Joseph's Angel of Mercy."

About a year later, the *Star* ran a story about a nurse who had founded a community health care center dedicated to serving children and adolescents.[31] The nurse, Ruth Ewert, had identified a glaring lack of adolescent health care services. So she raised the money to found a center to provide health care to adolescents. Instead of reflecting her knowledge, courage, and persistence, the headline introduced her as an "Angel in Our Midst." The article's subhead invited the reader to "meet Ruth Ewert, kind, gentle and a hero to all those whose lives she's touched."[32]

One of the major effects of this feedback loop is that it reinforces traditional gender dichotomies in which doctors, the knowledge workers, save lives, while nurses give comfort and kindness. In the spring of 2003, the *New York Times* Health Science section ran an article on the problem of premature births. The article featured a photograph of a nurse taking care of a sick baby in a neonatal intensive care unit. The caption read: "Cheryl Rolston, a nurse, tends to a small baby after a feeding." Although nurses and doctors together save these sick babies, the pull quote made it clear who the *Times* considered the most important player on the stage. "Doctors," it read, "can save most premature babies, but they haven't found a way to stop premature births." From its title to its captions and pull quotes, the article made it seem that only doctors are curious about the causes of prematurity and that they are the only ones that save sick babies.[33]

Given the social script, it is not surprising that patients who have survived because of nursing care also seem unable to recognize the knowledge and skill it embodies. In his book *Still Me*, the actor Christopher Reeve went into great detail describing the extraordinary activities of the doctors who saved his life after his equestrian accident. Of his ICU nurses, he had only this to say: "The nurses were so gentle. I still remember their sweet southern voices, trying to strike the correct balance between being sympathetic and being straightforward. One morning a favorite nurse, Joni, arranged for me to be taken up on the roof of the hospital to watch the sunrise."[34]

Four years later, Reeve published another book, *Nothing Is Impossible*, in which he details his long journey toward what he hopes will be recovery. With arduous effort, he did, in fact, do what some considered to be impossible: move his little finger. In this book, he revisited his accident and his time in the hospital. The nurses who cared for Reeve would probably be quite amazed to learn that he attributed their many contributions to doctors. "The critical care," he writes, "was nothing short of miraculous. Dr. John Jane—arguably one of the best neurosurgeons in the world—achieved the nearly impossible feat of reattaching the base of my skull to my spinal column with wire, titanium, and bone grafted from my hip. Under his watchful eye, a team of internists and pulmonologists cured me of ulcers and pneumonia."[35]

And later, nurses might be even more surprised to see themselves further demoted from clinicians to adolescent family members when he comments, "I was like a child and the doctors seemed like parents, while the nurses became older brothers and sisters."[36]

This feedback loop has also influenced one of the most expensive of the contemporary campaigns designed to address the nursing shortage. The Johnson & Johnson company has spent over $20 million on a campaign to support nursing and change its public image. With the help of nurse advisers, it has produced TV spots, promotional brochures, and a recruitment video in which nurses talk about their work and a video in which patients talk about the importance of nursing. They insisted it would make nurses feel proud of their work and at the same time transform how the public and even physicians view nursing.[37]

The company has broadcast its messages nationally and internationally on TV coverage of events like the 2002 Winter Olympics and has distributed eight million pieces of literature about nurses' work. The campaign's TV ads are accompanied by voice-overs and a sound track. The first image that appears on the screen is a female nurse who says, "The art and science of medicine and awesome nursing care can produce miracles." The sound track has the following ditty:

> There are some who live for caring with all they have to give
> There are some who have comfort to share
> They dare to care
> They dare to cry
> They dare to feel
> They dare to try
> They dare to be, at the end of the day,
> More than they were the day before.
> There are some who find their treasure inside a grateful smile
> There are some who will always be there.
> There are some who make the journey to find out who they are
> There are some who have the courage to care
> There are some who dare to care.[38]

In the Johnson & Johnson four-minute recruitment video, a male nurse states:

Being a nurse is all about holding someone's hand. Being a nurse is about giving a really good shot to a six-year-old who's terrified. It's about putting an ice pack and making it better on someone . . . or getting the wrinkles out of the back of a sheet that's causing someone to be uncomfortable who has to lay on the bed. They don't have any other place to go. They have to be there. And sometimes, you know, just rubbing someone's back is the answer to all their prayers.[39]

The jingle that accompanies the video on patients' perspectives of nursing includes the following lines:

> You're always there when someone needs you
> You work your magic quietly
> You're not in it for the glory
> The care you give comes naturally
> You take my hand
> Touch my life
> When I need you.[40]

One is struck by the similarity of these messages to those that Hallmark has on its Nurses Week cards. "What is a nurse?" one of its 2002 Nurses

Week cards asks: "A nurse," Hallmark replies, "is a special person, an angel in disguise, with tenderness in every touch, and caring watchful eyes."

Virtue 2: The Need for Knowledge and the End to Angels

As nurses in the twenty-first century come under increasing pressure to concretely connect nursing practice and patient outcomes, it is difficult to understand why nursing and nurses appear to have such a limited vocabulary when talking about and promoting the importance of their work. When women in other professions have moved from virtue to knowledge, why has this framing of nursing as a virtuous profession been so consistent? Even more difficult to understand is why, when there is now a great deal of data to document the critical importance of nursing to patient care, nursing groups make so little use of it. The most logical answer to this question is that nurses feel they gain something from this focus on virtue. One reason nurses may rely so heavily on this virtue script is that many believe this is their only legitimate source of status, respect, and self-esteem. For the past 150 years nurses have been told that medicine and physicians have more scientific knowledge and skill than they do. For over a century, nursing knowledge has been dismissed as "mere skill" or "tedious drudge work" that does not require the kind of "special knowledge" that the physician has mastered.[41] Deprived of the status and respect and self-esteem that flow from "discipline-specific cognitive-skills," nurses have been taught that the only way they can gain social respect is by being considered the most devoted, altruistic, and trustworthy members of the health care team.

The feedback loop we have described guarantees that nurses receive a great deal of public—and medical—support for following this script. Like the powerless nurse in the Medical University of South Carolina brochure, nurses consistently report that community members, along with patients and family members, thank them for their altruism as well as for the fact that they do work that many people find emotionally difficult. In our interviews with journalists and members of the public, nurses are constantly lauded for doing "a thankless" job, for being so "devoted," and for doing "something I could never do." Unless one specifically probes, rarely do the compliments nurses receive emphasize the knowledge, competence, and clinical judgment of the nurse.

Opinion polls paid for by nursing organizations reflect the same public support for the moral aspects of nursing. Highly publicized polls conducted in North America by Harris, Gallup, and the Canadian Polara, for example, give nurses very high marks for being more ethical, honest, and

trustworthy than doctors or, for that matter, members of many other occupation. When it comes to knowledge work, ratings of nurses, however,
plummet. When the Harris organization asked respondents whether they
would consult a nurse on a variety of health care issues about which nurses
clearly have great expertise, those who thought nurses were ethical and
honest apparently also believed they had only the most limited knowledge
and would not ask them questions about women's health, osteoporosis, or
sexually transmitted diseases.[42]

Given the persistence of institutional restrictions on nurses, it is also understandable that so many focus on their virtues. Nurses have told Gordon
that they are routinely chastised if they convey "medical" information to
patients, speak to the media on medical treatment or research, or advise
politicians and policymakers about "medical policy," in which they
nonetheless, play a critical role. They are not, however, penalized if they
talk about their caring, advocacy or their holistic or humanistic role. Thus, a
focus on virtue allows nursing a voice, albeit a limited one, in the public
discussion about health care. As they were in the past, physicians today,
like the medical director of the Hospital of the Medical University of South
Carolina, are more than willing to show their public appreciation for nurses
who play the right role amplifying "by their extended bedside presence the
value of our (physicians') brief daily patient encounters."

Toward a Knowledge Script

Sentimental and moralistic framings of the profession helped nurses
navigate the path from the nineteenth-century patriarchal home and family
to the hospital workplace and deal with the burgeoning medical profession. We have argued that over its long history, and particularly during its
nineteenth-century modernization, nursing was constructed as a gendered
moral practice with nurses depicted as "virtue" not "knowledge" workers.

Although, much has changed for professional women in the twentieth
century, nurses continue to rely on religious, moral, and sentimental sym-
bols and rhetoric—images of hearts, angels, touching hands, and appeals
based on diffuse references to closeness, intimacy, and making a difference.
Indeed, this moral framing appears to be a fundamental part of nurses'
claim to social legitimacy, as they assert their superior connection to patients and position themselves as the humanizing presence in an increasingly impersonal health care system. Thus, efforts to craft an image of the
"new nurse" continue to reflect and reinforce a central, enduring problematic for the profession: the often unacknowledged legacy of the nineteenth-
century reform of nursing.

When women had few social, legal, or economic rights, virtue was their trump card. Nurses have played the virtue card for 150 years, and during certain periods it helped them overcome considerable barriers. The persistent recourse to what we term the "virtue script" has, however, serious consequences for contemporary nursing. It may even discourage the right kind of nursing candidate from considering a career. Someone interested in combining caring with intellectual and scientific challenges would be likely to reject the traditional constellation of moral and ethical framings of the nurse. Finally, the virtue script undermines nurses' ability to help the public understand why researchers find that patient recovery—indeed their very lives—depends on adequate numbers of registered nurses. This inability to articulate the importance of nursing in the current climate of economic rationalism threatens the viability of nursing practice.

Today, as nurses are asked to justify their existence and describe their central importance to quality health care to hospital and health care managers, insurers, health care policymakers, politicians, and journalists, the virtue strategy is clearly not working. The public's belief that nurses do not have relevant medical expertise, the reluctance of journalists to turn to nurses as sources of health care news, and the fact that so many women view nursing as a lower-status profession because it is dominated by women indicates the failure of the virtue script to solve the problem of public respect for nursing.

When repeated in recruitment brochures and campaigns, appeals to virtue are unlikely to help people understand what nurses really do and how much knowledge and skill they need to do it. If these ads do attract people to nursing, one has to ask what kind of people they are. Will they be people interested only in sentimental work, who will thus be surprised to discover how tough and intellectually challenging nurses' work really is, and how little it resembles the Hallmark card fantasy? Similarly, one has to ask whether these appeals discourage candidates who want to combine caring for others with intellectual stimulation and deepening cognitive challenges. One has to also question whether these virtue appeals will attract more men into nursing.

While Johnson & Johnson and other organizations that sponsor virtue-based recruitment ads insist that they are attracting new candidates to nursing, the question that must be also researched is whether these candidates remain at the bedside, that is, in those areas of nursing that are so plagued by shortages. Preliminary reports, like those published in the United States and Great Britain, suggest that appeals to virtue may have a boomerang effect, leading new nurses into a revolving door, which they quickly exit once they discover the realities of hospital nursing duties and working conditions. The crisis in recruitment and, most critically, the retention of nurses demands that the value of nursing work, as opposed to the sentimental valuing of nurses, be made clear to the public and employers.

Finally, appeals to the moral value of nursing make it difficult for nurses to defend their work in a period of cost-cutting. When nurses argue that they are caring, holistic, humanistic virtue workers, their claims are generally dismissed by hospital administrators as mere sentiment, a luxury the hospital can no longer afford. For example, in her chapter on the dismantling of the once-powerful nursing department at Boston's Beth Israel Deaconess Medical Center, sociologist Dana Beth Weinberg explains that nurses' appeals to "humanism" and the "nurse-patient relationship" fell entirely on deaf ears when administrators wanted to save money by cutting nursing staff. In the absence of arguments that made concrete connections between nurses' knowledge and patient outcomes, a model of nursing care that had been built over decades was dismantled in a matter of months. As one hospital administrator recently told Suzanne Gordon, "We are not hiring humanists in the hospital these days."

Consider, for example, how this focus on virtue could be recast and how a truly new image of nursing, one that focuses on knowledge, could be produced. In 1997 the British Columbia Nurses Union produced a campaign to explain the importance of nursing to the public. In one ad, a nurse is standing smiling at a patient's bedside as he is about to begin eating his hospital meal. The ad copy reads:

> He thinks he's having a conversation about the hospital Jell-O. She's actually midway through about 100 assessments. In the seconds it takes to reach the bedside, a Registered Nurse will have made over 100 assessments.
>
> Any one of which could mean the difference between recovery and tragedy.
>
> Take away direct patient care from Registered Nurses and vital knowledge affecting the health of the patient is lost.
>
> Nurses are doing vital work. It's that simple. While rethinking our regional health care system, it is vital to strengthen the role of Registered Nurses, the most comprehensively trained nurses in the system.
>
> Registered Nurses are not an adjunct to our evolving health care system, they are at the very hub of it. Making sure they keep direct patient contact is critical to the quality of our health care system.
>
> While they may not be specialists in green Jell-O, when it comes to health care, Registered Nurses are irreplaceable.

Finally, consider how Gordon has rewritten the copy for the Johnson & Johnson campaign:

Being a nurse is about making sure a patient doesn't develop a fatal complication after surgery. It's about paying attention to the smallest but most significant details. Like smoothing out the wrinkles on a sheet so a patient doesn't develop an excruciating and costly bedsore. Sometimes by sitting and talking to someone, I find out the most important things, like whether patients understand how to take their medications, whether they have support at home, and whether they are frightened and anxious.

If the nursing profession is to be successful in attracting new recruits who will stay at the bedside, if it is to be able to change the working conditions and pay scales that now discourage long-term nurse retention, and if it is to fashion a new image, it must move from a focus on virtue to one on knowledge.

2

When Little Things Are Big Things

The Importance of Relationships for Nurses' Professional Practice

Dana Beth Weinberg

What do nurses do? As a novice sociologist with no background in nursing, I had only vague notions about what nurses do when I began conducting fieldwork at Beth Israel Deaconess Medical Center (BIDMC) in 1999. My interest as a researcher was in exploring the effects of restructuring on frontline employees. Beth Israel Hospital had recently been through a merger with New England Deaconess Hospital, and the ill effects on the hospital's care were regularly featured in the *Boston Globe*. Due to the urging of my mentor, who had recently been a BIDMC patient and was struck by the nurses' plight, I chose to study the effects of the merger and other large-scale changes at the hospital on nurses, the quintessential front line. I wanted to understand how things like a merger and budget cuts might affect nurses' daily work and what the implications might be for nurses and patients. The product of my research, *Code Green: Money-Driven Hospitals and the Dismantling of Nursing*, explained how hospital restructuring was contributing to our nation's critical shortage of nurses.[1] My work documented how hospitals, in response to financial concerns, were inadvertently changing nurses' work in ways that made nursing a less attractive career and compromised nurses' ability to provide high-quality patient care.

Understanding change first required an understanding of the work itself. As I observed nurses at work and interviewed them and hospital administrators, my ignorance about nursing forced me repeatedly to ask the fundamental question, "What do nurses do?" I had no idea how essential this question would be to understanding the effects of restructuring on nurses at that particular hospital. Nor did I realize at the time how important the nurses' answers would be for explaining why, despite nurses' objections, particular changes were so prevalent in financially struggling U.S. hospitals for the past decade.

In answer to my questions and those of many administrators and consultants, nurses' descriptions of their work often emphasized developing relationships with patients, rather than the professional activities I witnessed as I shadowed them. The lack of consistency between the nurses' abstract, relationship-oriented accounts and my daily observations of therapeutic activities that patients depend on was puzzling, particularly since the nurses at Beth Israel Deaconess Medical Center were a highly seasoned and professional bunch. More than puzzling, however, these responses became pivotal in the unfolding story of the dismantling of this famous nursing service. As hospital administrators panicked about the hospital's finances, they introduced a series of changes meant to streamline work and reduce costs. Although the nurses were becoming increasingly dissatisfied and suffering from burnout, they failed to articulate restructuring's negative effects and advocate for themselves and their patients. In a pattern increasingly prevalent in hospitals across the country, nurses were quietly choosing to leave the bedside and the profession rather than challenge financially motivated changes that endangered nurses and patients.

Relationships with Patients

For over a quarter century, Beth Israel had worked hard to build one of the most recognized and studied professional nursing programs in the world. Among nurses, the hospital had gained a reputation as a good place to work. In the 1980s when other hospitals struggled with nursing shortages, Beth Israel had no difficulty attracting highly skilled nurses and even ran a series of advertisements emphasizing the quality of their nursing service as a distinctive advantage of care at the hospital. "It's the nurses" was the slogan. Their nursing service distinguished Beth Israel from the other teaching hospitals in Boston and earned it the reputation of being "Harvard with a heart."

Although nurses received kudos from the hospital and the community for being attentive to patients, what distinguished nursing at Beth Israel was not that nurses there were nice but that they were highly professional. With Joyce Clifford at the head of the nursing department, Beth Israel had gained national and international recognition as a pioneer in developing and nurturing a professional practice model for nursing. For years, Beth Israel hired only nurses with four-year degrees, encouraged nurses to go back to school for graduate degrees, and provided a great deal of in-house education. Beth Israel's professional practice model revolved around the concept of primary nursing, a system that involved the same nurse caring for the same patient from admission to discharge. In its formulation, primary nursing elevated the professional status of nurses by defining even so-called mundane tasks as part of a complicated process of evaluating patients, planning and implementing their nursing care, coordinating that care with other members of the care team, and continually reassessing the efficacy of interventions through a serious program of research. Nurses, rather than nurses' aides or other less-skilled personnel, provided almost all aspects of nursing care. Through twenty-four-hour accountability and continuity of care, the system enabled the nurse to familiarize herself with her patients' unique needs and tailor their care.

For years, reference to these nurse-patient relationships empowered Beth Israel nurses, enhancing the nursing department's prestige and the central role of nurses in patient care. While doctors still inevitably called the shots, the nurses' opinions mattered, and nurses acted as strong advocates for patients.

The Need to Defend Nursing

With the budget cuts that plagued hospitals nationwide in the 1990s, something changed. To survive under managed care and in an environment rife with hospital mergers, in 1996 the Beth Israel Hospital decided it had to merge with its neighbor, the New England Deaconess Hospital, to become Beth Israel Deaconess Medical Center. In 1999, in the middle of the most turbulent period of this merger, I spent over nine months shadowing nurses and interviewing hospital administrators and staff about the changes taking place and their effect on nursing. The merger had cost an enormous amount of money and caused many unintended problems. With these, as well as a decline in reimbursements, the hospital faced a dire financial situation. BIDMC's financial crisis precipitated an emphasis on cost-cutting and streamlining measures, such as shortening the length of stay and reducing support services. Like nurses in other hospitals across the United States, Beth Israel nurses were asked to defend their position in the hospital. Like other institutions that were restructuring at this time, the hospital brought in outside consultants who turned a critical eye to the hospital's budget. They targeted nursing as an area for reductions and presented the nursing service with a series of questions becoming commonplace in hospitals across the country: Couldn't nurses care for more or sicker patients with fewer resources and in less time? Couldn't they work with unlicensed nursing assistants? Couldn't they pick up some of the small tasks performed by support personnel, like blood draws and patient transport?

Once the darlings of the hospital, the nurses suddenly found that they needed to advocate not only for their patients but for themselves, their practice model, and their department. Although they shared a growing concern that patient care at this highly respected hospital was becoming unsafe, the Beth Israel nurses floundered when confronted with the need to explain their work and mount a successful internal campaign to protect the resources needed to provide the high-quality nursing care that had been the hospital's trademark

Despite the frantic, backbreaking pace that I witnessed from floor nurses as I followed them day after day, in my interviews they provided weak accounts of how the shortened length of stay or reduced support services affected their work. In general, the highly educated and experienced nurses I interviewed did not present concrete details of what nurses do and how restructuring prevented them from doing it. More often than not, nurses instead lamented a diminished ability to know patients as people and develop relationships with them. For example, one veteran nurse complained, "Now, we have more patients and they are sicker. They don't stay here as long. . . . It's much more fast paced." She emphasized the negative effect that these changes were having on patient care: "There isn't room for the personal care that they used to get. There isn't time to get to know your patients as people as much because you don't have a lot of chitchat time anymore." The main difference in her practice, she told me, was

> how personal you are, how if you walk in they know your name right away. You are able to give a piece of yourself. There isn't time to give a piece of yourself anymore. . . . It's a one-way relationship now. It used to be give and take. You'd sit on the bed with a ninety-eight-year-old man and say, "So what did you do to live this long. What's your secret?" I don't have time to do that anymore.

In a separate interview, another nurse similarly described the situation:

> It's just you don't get the time to spend with people, . . . spend some time listening to their concerns and [listening] to their complaints or whatever it is that they need to talk about. . . . On a day when it's so busy and all I'm doing is quickly jumping in asking some questions, . . . [doing] my whole assessment, putting in an IV, drawing blood, and running out of the room so that I can type it up into the computer so they can be admitted, you don't feel like you've done what you could do for somebody.

Commenting on the same set of changes, another nurse lamented:

There's no personal touch. Or there's not even really a lot of compassion for these people who are acutely ill. That stuff really makes me feel that it's not what it used to be, in a very disgusted sort of way. It doesn't take a whole lot to make someone feel special or to sit with them for fifteen minutes and say, "What do you need?"

This kind of language was used at every level of the nursing hierarchy. When asked to justify nursing expenses, which the hospital was eager to slash, frontline nurses, nurse managers, and nurse executives retreated to a quality of care argument steeped in this language of relationships. To present the evidence, they adopted the language of the nurses I interviewed: Nurses do not have enough time for "little things," for that "little bit extra," to "get the patients comfortable, to give "personal care," to "know your patients as people," to "develop relationships," to "do what you could for somebody," to "make someone feel special."

Despite the carefully nurtured professionalism of the Beth Israel nurses, most failed to connect explicitly how time to do the "little things" enables nurses to do the big things—assess patients, monitor their progress, plan care, and carry out medical interventions. Had nurses been able to describe the problems with their practice in the professional terms of therapeutic activities—in terms of what nurses *do*—they would have been able to argue that hospitals could not afford to do without the "little things." In fact, they would have been able to convincingly argue, as Gordon does, that when it comes to the care of the sick, there is no such thing as a little thing.[2]

Rather than talking about their diminished ability to do their jobs and citing the growing number of studies that documented the potentially dire consequences for patients[3] the nurses spoke instead about loss of relationships:

So as far as my job, I don't like my job as much as I used to. I used to be rewarded by the relationships that I developed with people over time. Now, with this quick turnaround, you don't develop the same relationships. You do your best and you have to be satisfied that you are doing the best that you can because you're not doing as good as you used to.

In the interviews I conducted, I found it extremely difficult to get nurses to move beyond the rhetoric of relationships and describe how restructuring might be changing what they actually do.

Nurses' focus on personal relationships prevented them from describing how care was being threatened when restructuring deprived them of enough time to know patients, and it bore little resemblance to the daily practice I observed. Although many nurses equated developing relationships with patients with providing care, none of them was actively trying to "get to know" their patients in the sense of cultivating a friendship. In the nine months I followed nurses at Beth Israel, I did not see them make friends with patients or indulge in unproductive chitchat. The very skilled and experienced nurses I observed did not compellingly explain that gathering, interpreting, exchanging, and acting on information about patients was their stock and trade.

Consider the typical pattern of daily activities I witnessed while shadowing nurses at BIDMC. At the beginning of the shift, a nurse would receive reports on her (very few nurses were male) patients from the outgoing shift. She would familiarize herself with patients' names and the type of care and treatment they might receive over the course of the day. Different medical and surgical teams made their rounds on the units, and more than one team at a time might supervise a patient's care. Nurses coordinated the orders and instructions from all of these teams. Since nurses did not usually make rounds with the teams, this coordination often entailed tracking down the physicians in charge of their patients either in person or by phone.

After a nurse finished receiving a verbal report and reviewing notes on her patients—each with a unique set of problems and needs—she checked in with the patients. Sometimes a quick darting in and out of a patient's room sufficed. Other times the initial visit lasted well beyond a half hour, as the nurse dealt with complicated medical issues. In what seemed like constant motion, nurses juggled numerous tasks simultaneously. Nurses worked nonstop changing IV bags, administering pills, taking vital signs, helping patients to the commode—all while chatting with the patient and sometimes the patient's family. The nurses fielded questions from anxious family members and explained medications and self-care to patients and their families. The nurses also coordinated admissions and discharge of patients from their units. The preparation and paperwork involved could be time consuming, with one discharge requiring up to three hours of work as nurses contacted physicians, case managers, families, and insurance companies.

My persistent efforts to uncover how restructuring might affect what nurses do helped me decode what nurses meant by "knowing patients." Getting to know patients was an integral part of nurses' daily activities. However, this "knowing" did not involve some superficial friendliness or attempt to develop personal intimacy. Knowing patients meant knowing about a patient's medical needs and progress, not their personal stories and dreams. Knowing the patient involved learning about the physical and emotional dimensions of a patient's illness, finding out how the patient responded to treatment and managed complex medication regimens, and discerning what resources the patient would need to cope with their illness and treatment regimens once they left the hospital. Knowing the patient required familiarity with their medical record, with the care plans of other care providers, with the patient's current physical and emotional state, and with the patient's home situation. Knowing the patient was a professional, not a personal, activity; nurses did not share their own personal information with patients in a mutual process of getting to know one another. Relationships with patients, I deduced through my observations, were not personal relationships but therapeutic ones.

During the period of my fieldwork, I conducted interviews with thirty-four nurses and seven focus groups with a total of thirty-eight nurses. The problem of not having enough time to know patients emerged in almost every conversation, but most of the nurses in my study did a poor job articulating the therapeutic content of "knowing the patient." In contrast, in those rare instances when the nurses I interviewed focused on what they actually do, the importance of knowing patients as a primary therapeutic tool became apparent. "It's hard to document and to show what it is you do when you walk into a room and say hello to a patient," an emergency room nurse told me. She illustrated how what might easily be described as getting to know a patient or developing a relationship was really about establishing a fundamental therapeutic groundwork. "Anybody," she said, "can walk into a room and say hello," but nurses were doing something "that's different." The difference, she explained, has to do with assessing and evaluating patients:

> In an emergency room the whole thing is about evaluating them. . . . We don't know what's wrong with them. . . . Our patients are complete strangers, and they came to the emergency room because they believed they were having an emergency. Some of them are, and some of them aren't. But you need somebody with them who can determine which is which.

The nurse possessed the professional knowledge to tell the difference. Doing "some of the task things," she explained, allowed nurses the opportunity to "to talk to your patient, get a better sense of what's going on with them, interview your patient, talk to the family that's in there, and sort out what's going on and get a better feel for the patient."

Another nurse offered a similar account of what nurses are doing when they perform basic tasks. She faulted her colleagues, "We've really not been good about making people understand what's going on. And part of it is that nurses, themselves, don't know what they're doing." She explained,

"You ask them what they were doing and they'll say, 'Oh, I was just check-ing on a patient.'" Such a response diminishes the concrete contributions that nurses make to the quality of care and limits nurses' ability to explain how less time with patients might threaten patient care. As this veteran nurse pointed out, "Just checking on a patient is an extremely complicated thing. And most of it you're doing unconsciously. . . . Because if you're looking for response to illness, which is what nursing is doing, then those responses are very subtle and very wide ranging." She explained with a more concrete example, "You evaluate patients by working with them. What happens when you ask them to put their arm out? Did they put their arm out? Did they seem to understand you? Are they paying attention? Are they restless? Well, you can't tell those things by flitting in and out of the room in two minutes." According to these two nurses, performing the busy task work provided the opportunity to observe and interact with patients that enabled nurses to assess them. While many nursing tasks did not al-ways require a great degree of skill to perform, they provided a vehicle for gathering rich information about patients. Nurses' skills, training, and clin-ical judgment then enabled them to assemble these disparate pieces of in-formation in a meaningful way.

In a different interview, a third nurse explained to me the therapeutic importance of her knowledge of patients. "You've had them every night for five nights," she explained, while the doctors "don't know boo about them. . . . And how many times will an intern say, 'What do you think we should do? You know them. What do you think?'" The nurse's answer to the intern's question has little to do with the personal friendliness between the nurse and her patient. Rather, it requires an understanding of the pa-tient's treatment history and responses to various interventions: "I'll say, 'Well, last time this happened, this is what we did. It didn't work; so then we did this. Why don't we do this?'" In this example, the nurse's knowl-edge of her patient helped her advocate for a potentially more effective treatment option. Another nurse, providing similar insight into the thera-peutic importance of knowing patients, explained, "If you don't take it on yourself to understand the patient's situation—what the patient's problems are—you won't develop a plan to do something about them."

For nurses, relationships with patients are instrumental, a means to an end. Nurses need time with patients in order to evaluate, plan, and per-form their care. While nurses knew this implicitly, their discussion did not often differentiate between the therapeutic relationships necessary to de-liver care and personal relationships. The limited time with patients jeop-ardized the therapeutic relationships through which nurses gather, ex-change, and act on relevant information about their patients. In short, restructuring, by reducing nurses' time with patients, strained nurses' ability to provide safe care.

Unless I probed, however, nurses rarely broke the code. They seemed to automatically default to relationship talk when asked about their work. Not only did they do this in interviews with me but also with administrators making budget decisions. I, however, had the time and inclination to push them to examine the disconnect between what they said and what they actually did. Administrators, in contrast, were not aware that they needed to decipher what nurses meant by "knowing patients" and "developing relationships." Had they known, they still may not have been willing to do the necessary investigative work.

But when nurses relied on pictures of personal intimacy to plead the case that restructuring was harming patient care, the language of personal connection undercut their challenge to the market view of the hospital. Confronted with these pictures of personal intimacy, hospital administrators easily dismissed time with patients as a luxury they cannot afford. How could doing "little things" be a priority for a hospital hemorrhaging money?

When the Problem Is Framed as Personal

On hearing accounts from nurses about their not having enough time with patients to develop relationships, administrators zeroed in, not on nurses' concerns about quality but on their lost "sources of gratification." An administrator involved in planning hospital restructuring stated:

> In the delivery of health care, [health care professionals] increasingly are pushed toward being mere "functionaries." . . . That takes out in your own personal experience, especially those who practiced over time; it takes out what you probably value as part of your practice. There will be another generation . . . coming in who could just take this on, and you don't know what's missing, and you'll find . . . other sources of gratification. . . . Part of the bitterness here, quite frankly, has to do with the aging workforce who remember . . . the good old days.

One nurse administrator, for example, opined that the problem had less to do with poor quality of care than it did with learning to accept change: "[Time with patients] is a big issue. A very big issue. Some of that I think is very legitimate, and some of it is really needing to learn how to change. We just can't go back to before. . . . That's the loss that people are feeling. It's a loss that all clinicians are feeling. Nurses are in a very hard and unforgiving environment right now." To the extent that relationships represented a now absent source of job satisfaction for nurses, nurses' concerns about not hav-ing enough time with patients could be dismissed as an unwillingness to accept "necessary" change rather than warnings about problems with care.

As this administrator's comments well indicate, the personal relation-ship frame made it seem that nurses' personal satisfaction, rather than es-sential therapeutic time, was being eliminated by the hospital to save money. The loss of time with patients, then, became a personal problem, not a professional one that compromised patient safety. Such a personal problem, moreover, had a personal solution. "I think it's also up to the per-son," a nurse told me, "because it's in your hands. Like you can not eat your lunch and spend more time with the patient, if it's needed. . . . Like people have control over it. You can be . . . spending time with them like if you really, really want to do it." She accused some of her colleagues of using lack of time "as a cop-out to not do things." Many of the nurses I in-terviewed shared this view that spending time with patients was a matter of personal choice, and they frequently faulted themselves if they did not have enough time.

Rather than confront a system for denying nurses what they need to care for patients, nurses instead placed increasingly greater demands on them-selves. Nurses went to personal extremes to increase the time they could spend with patients. Nurses sped up their work during the day; they jogged, rather than walked, up and down the hospital corridors. Many worked eight or more hours at a stretch without taking a break, and many went almost whole shifts without eating or relieving themselves. "It's not unusual for me to work a twelve-hour shift and not be able to eat lunch till four or five o'clock. We have days like that too, where you can't stop. And there are a number of days where you go without eating at all," a nurse told me. "There are days you don't eat lunch until three or four o'clock, starting at 7 a.m. There are days you try to get to the bathroom by three, lit-erally." In addition to denying themselves breaks, nurses also stayed late to complete work, rather than ignore the "little things" for which they lacked time during their hectic shifts. Nurses were clear that the decision of whether or not to stay rested with the individual nurse: "It's really personal preference."

In addition, a number of nurses reduced their work hours from full time to part time or did per diem work. Linking this trend to nurses' regular de-cisions to stay late, a nurse explained that she never worked a regular forty-hour week: "forty hours is baloney; it's sixty hours, seventy hours. . . . Part-time is easier for me. . . . If I get out at one in the morning [instead of at eleven], that's okay. It's one shift." Working on a part-time or per diem basis enabled nurses to work more hours on fewer shifts without suffering the burnout that would result from doing a full-time schedule with so many additional hours.

If "doing the little things" is seen as a "personal preference" or a "source of gratification" and not a professional necessity, it does not explain why nurses went to such extremes, risking burnout, to increase their time with patients. It did not make sense that nurses, with lives and families outside of the hospital, would receive so much satisfaction from their personal connections with patients that they willingly worked "a twelve-hour shift every day, when they're getting paid for eight hours."

The pervasiveness of these rather extensive self-sacrificing practices pointed to a fundamental problem in care delivery at BIDMC, not a crisis in nurses' personal satisfaction. The reason that nurses sped up their work and stayed late had little to do with personal relationships and everything to do with providing professional nursing care. They overworked, not so that they could enjoy greater job satisfaction, but so that they could accomplish basic patient care that met their professional standards. They skipped bathroom breaks, not because they wanted to make friends with their patients, but because they worried that their patients could die, have preventable complications, or otherwise suffer if they did not receive needed care.

By government regulation, nurses are responsible for the care their patients receive. The public depends on nurses to ensure that patients receive appropriate care, as determined by a professional trained and licensed to make that determination. This responsibility is not a matter of individual commitment but of professional accountability. Nurses at BIDMC internalized this mandate. When a nurse failed to deliver the care she thought her patients needed, she called herself a "bad nurse." As an outsider, I found this self-blame bewildering. Why not in this same situation call BIDMC a "bad hospital"? After all, nurses are hospital employees, and the hospital, not the individual nurse, determines a nurse's work conditions. Nurses do not decide how many patients they are going to care for on a given shift, how sick those patient will be or what types of problems they will have, or what resources will be at their disposal for providing care. Hospital administrators, however, do control the budgets and policies that determine these factors. With restructuring, hospital administrators reduced the resources available to nurses. Nurses got the message, "Make do with less. Do what you normally do or try to do what you normally do, but do it with fewer resources and do it with less staff."

In order to maintain a level of quality care that met nurses' professional standards, nurses tried to work longer and harder to temper the consequences of the poorer standard of care produced by the hospital's new budget and policies. As resources diminished, nurses sacrificed increasing amounts of personal time and energy in an attempt to cram even more into their eight-hour shifts and stayed late to give the care they could not give during their shifts.

Administrators (and even some nurses) claimed, however, that spending time with patients contributed to nurses' satisfaction, not to patient outcomes. In this way, they were able to belittle the idea that lacking time with patients was a legitimate source of complaint in a financially struggling hospital. This struck me as quite strange, particularly since a large body of work in the social sciences links worker satisfaction and burnout to performance outcomes. What might be the impact of burnout and dissatisfaction on patient care? Additionally, several studies linking nurse staffing to patient outcomes were beginning to emerge, and yet nurses and nurse administrators failed to point to these scientific findings as they argued about the need for better staffing and support. Whether or not administrators wanted to address the issue of how nurses' satisfaction and burnout might affect patient care in the short term, there was a national story emerging about long-term effects. In particular, the impending nursing shortage was already creating a great deal of buzz nationwide. Beth Israel Hospital's nursing service had initially gained recognition for its ability to attract and retain nurses, even during the national nursing shortage in the 1980s. Yet, a quarter of the nurses I studied were intent on leaving their jobs in the next year, making Beth Israel no different from other hospitals in the country.[4] Nurses could easily have pointed to the potential consequences for the hospital's reputation and its future ability to provide high quality patient care. They did not.

What made this response even more poignant was the growing activity by nurses' unions in the greater-Boston area and across the country. Unlike other nurses, both in Boston—in fact, just across the street at Brigham and Women's Hospital—and nationwide, who were publicly protesting cuts in nursing staff and unmanageable workloads, the Beth Israel nurses did not go public with their complaints. The nurses at BIDMC treated the problem of time with patients, nurses' burnout, and their intention to quit as a matter strictly internal to the hospital and personal for the individual nurse. Even though the nurses I interviewed cried about the changes to their jobs and warned about the threat to patients, when confronted with the option of going public, they backed down. They did not join the broader debate that was taking place around them and even seemed unaware of this larger national conversation and potential sources of support. When asked about the potential of unions to help them, nurses pooh-poohed the idea and never contacted the media or joined protests. They viewed unions as incompatible with the professionalism so strongly emphasized by their nursing model; unions were for wage workers, they reasoned, not *professional* nurses. Even as their model of nursing was being dismantled, they refused to seek outside support to help them make the argument about patient safety that on their own they were ineffective in making. Perhaps cowed by the accusation that they were concerned only about their own satisfaction, the nurses at BIDMC failed to provide their administrators or the public with any evidence of the critical link between the quality of their work life and patient care.

Nurses' construction of their work as personal and relational, rather than professional, diminished the serious problem of not having enough time with patients. This personal construction enabled administrators to call "loss of time" a personal loss, rather than a clinical or quality of care loss. In addition, it drove nurses to see time with patients as a personal choice not a necessity for performing their professional work. Consequently, nurses repeatedly faulted themselves for poor care quality and pushed themselves to work harder, while hospital administrators maintained the illusion that nurses had the resources necessary to do their jobs.

As hospitals seek ways to maintain their financial footing in a turbulent health care market, they will continue to seek ways to restructure their organizations, work processes, and services. In order for nurses to protect themselves and patients, nurses must talk about what they actually do and how restructuring initiatives will affect that. This requires getting beyond the familiar aphorism, "Doctors cure and nurses care." An emphasis on relationships, disconnected from nurses' professional actions, does not communicate why nurses are vitally important to health care. Although the nurses I studied at BIDMC did not often draw the connection, my efforts uncovered the link between relationships with patients and care quality. It was indeed critical to have relationships with patients, but not the personal relationships so often invoked by Beth Israel nurses. Rather, the necessary relationships, and the ones being lost with restructuring, were the therapeutic interactions at the foundation of nurses' professional activities.

As a researcher, I had the time and tools to look beyond the surface. I had the opportunity to explore why nurses were going to personal extremes to preserve what at first glance appeared to be mere niceties and sources of satisfaction. I could spend time documenting and analyzing the effects of restructuring on nurses' daily activities and the mysterious disconnect between nurses' relationship talk and their actual activities.

If nurses want to protect themselves and patient care, they cannot wait for interested observers to figure out what is going on. Hospital administrators, consultants, and politicians will not expend the effort to decode and dissect nurses' relationship talk. Nurses need to be able to draw a vivid picture of how particular changes affect their work. The first step is to articulate what nurses as professionals do and why the little things are really big things.

3

Pride and Prejudice
Nurses' Struggle with Reasoned Debate

Diana J. Mason

"When nurses are referred to as angels, as sometimes happens in popular and professional literature, on television, and in advertising, it doesn't make me proud. . . . That so many nurses see nursing as a calling is a longstanding tradition that has nothing to do with the work we do. . . . I am a nurse. It is my job." So wrote Margaret C. Belcher, RN, BSN, CCRN, a nurse in the surgical-trauma intensive care unit at Tampa General Hospital, in a commentary published in the July 2004 issue of the *American Journal of Nursing*, of which I am the editor-in-chief.[1] In doing so, she unleashed an avalanche of mail from irate nurses who found her an embarrassment to the profession for suggesting that we eschew the worship of nursing as holy self-sacrifice in service of others.

After a few weeks of receiving a number of letters to the editor, almost all of which expressed outrage at her viewpoint, I shared them with Belcher via e-mail, noting that she had clearly touched a nerve. She wrote back telling me that she, too, had received similar e-mail and now regretted writing the piece. Most of the e-mail attacked her personally (as did many of the letters received in my office, though we delete personal attacks from letters we publish or simply don't publish them), and some called her unfit to be a nurse. We did publish four letters in the October issue of the journal, three of which articulated some reasoned disagreement with her position. I was dismayed and disappointed that my nursing colleagues would so contradict themselves—demonstrating that they are truly not angels after all—by attacking Belcher personally rather than simply disagreeing with her ideas. This experience so intimidated her that she decided it wiser to silence her voice than to continue to challenge the status quo.

Yet this response from readers did not surprise me. This was not my first experience with the problem of some nurses avoiding reasoned debate and assailing the messenger of difficult news rather than critiquing the message. On many occasions, I have borne the brunt of nurses' ad hominem attacks for editorials I had written that were designed to provoke debate on important issues confronting our profession. And I have been personally attacked for simply publishing the work of others that readers didn't like.

None has engendered the scale and depth of condemnation as something we published earlier in 2004. What was the offensive item? A poem. In the January issue we published a poem titled "Learning the Bones" by Shanna R. Germain that we knew would not sit well with some readers.[2] It had received high marks from reviewers, though several questioned how readers would respond to it. The fifteen-line poem portrays the musings of a student who is learning to navigate both her professional and personal life, including an affair with a detached, married lover, and coming to realize that personal life is harder than professional life. The editorial staff thought it important to be willing to tolerate some negative feedback from those uncomfortable with sexual matters, so we decided to "stretch," taking the risk to publish it.

Shortly after the poem was published, the mail began to pour in. And it poured and poured. Over the following months, we received over two hundred letters and pieces of e-mail. Nothing we had published since I became editor in chief of the journal in 1999 had generated more than twenty letters. Though we like mail at *AJN* and love to hear what readers think about what we're publishing, we were concerned that all of the early mail was opposed to our publishing the poem. Some writers asked, "What could you possibly have been thinking to publish this poem?" Some faculty said they were embarrassed to have their students see the poem and would no longer recommend that their students read *AJN*—this, even though the issue also included articles on such important topics as talking with patients and families about terminal illness, how to ask women about douching and discuss its dangers, and ten myths about Medicare. Others who wrote challenged my assertions in previous editorials that nurses needed to be proactive to stop media images of nurses that were demeaning, claiming that I had contributed to nursing's poor image by suggesting that nurses were adulterous. A number of readers said they were canceling their subscriptions to the journal.

I respond via e-mail or regular mail to almost every letter that the journal receives, in the belief that it will encourage readers who take the time to write to us to continue discussing and writing letters about what they read in the journal and elsewhere. I wrote personal replies to all the e-mail about the poem that came in. As the deluge continued, I began to use several standard replies (though I still personalized most of these). I eventually stopped responding to e-mail letters about it at all. The outrage about the poem found its way into chat rooms and onto e-mail subscription lists. Sentences from the e-mail I had written in response to the e-mail letters-to-the-editor were being posted to illustrate how unfit I was to be editor in chief of *AJN*. Subscription list users were encouraged to participate in a letter-writing campaign to me, the American Nurses Association (in 2004, *AJN* was the official journal of the ANA), and to Jay Lippincott, the president of Lippincott Williams & Wilkins, which owns and publishes *AJN*. I was alerted to this by a colleague who was on one of these subscriber lists and forwarded to me a posting from someone I did not know who berated me on the list, saying I was "a disgrace to the profession." She had done a Google search on me, taken statements I had made out of context and posted them on the list to illustrate how I was a destructive force for the profession and had to be stopped. Letters to Jay Lippincott called for my termination as editor in chief of the journal.

"Ah, the power of poetry," said Joy Jacobson, our managing editor. Indeed, but what was disturbing was the lack of thoughtful analysis of the poem by most who objected to it. I asked a respected nurse-poet, Cortney Davis, what she thought of the poem. She wrote a letter that we published, along with three pages of letters by others, in the April 2004 issue.[3] Her letter began, "I very much admire *AJN*'s courage in publishing 'Learning the Bones,' a poem that may well draw criticism from those who prefer poetry to be safe and sentimental."

"Safe and sentimental"—after months of being harangued, debased, and threatened, that's what I wanted life to be. I realized that, as Belcher later expressed, my fellow nurses had left me questioning the importance of risk taking and exploring new territory in my professional life. But I quickly realized that my colleagues' ad hominem responses were typical of a strand of contemporary nursing and were symptomatic of four conditions: a trend of avoiding reasoned debate on issues in politics and media in our society; the inadequacies of nursing education; a profession that is too often mired in oppressive group behavior, in which self-degradation prevails; and the emphasis on "self" in nursing.

Lack of Reasoned Debate in Society

Nurses are part of and reflect contemporary American society, where "talk back" and "talk over" television programs have replaced thoughtful exploration of important issues. The rise of Fox News, like many other news sources, has provided viewers with a polemical approach to the news of the day, providing one-sided discussions of issues. The message is that if you're not in our camp, you're a fool or part of the enemy camp. Our politics are replete with mudslinging attacks on candidates for public office and on policymakers. James Fallows has argued that it's easier for journalists to discuss the politics of an issue than the issue itself, leaving the public with few examples of reasoned discussions of the issues.[4] This is what nurses see around them, so why should they be any different?

Nursing Education

Nursing education also contributes to the problem. It is based on a punitive model of learning that originated in the church and the military. Although moving nursing education into the university has helped its discourse, my experience as an educator has shown me that relatively few nurse educators can tolerate nursing students who challenge their positions and teachings. We should be encouraging and rewarding respectful disagreement. Instead, students fear that speaking out may result in a poor grade or even failure, particularly in clinical courses, where the evaluation of performance is much more subjective than in the classroom. Where and how do nurses learn how to have reasoned debate? Where do they discuss how to challenge prevailing thought in respectful, objective ways? Rarely do they find this in nursing education, and they certainly do not find it in the workplace, where even unionized nurses often fear retaliation for speaking out about important issues such as conditions that jeopardize patient safety.

Oppressed Group Behavior

Particularly disturbing is nurses' inability to challenge the oppression and devaluation of nurses and patients that is prevalent in most health care settings. For years it's been clear to me that too many nurses are demeaned and disparaged at work. They feel powerless, so they exert their power over patients and one another. In response to some of the letters I received about Germain's poem, in which my commitment to nursing was belittled, I challenged the letter writers to demonstrate the same outspoken challenge and activism (since that was clearly how some on one subscriber list were viewing their letter-writing campaign) on issues of real importance to nursing and health care, for example, understaffing and mandatory overtime, or the growth in the number of uninsured people and children in poverty in this country. My angered response reflected my own dismay over what I believe is one of nursing's most challenging paradoxes. We know we have the potential to use our massive numbers to demand that society and our workplaces hold us in the regard that we believe we deserve, given our importance to the health care system and to the health of patients, but we are too often reluctant to take the actions needed to challenge the status quo in health care, and we tend to respond emotionally to challenges to the profession's status quo, despite knowing that we cannot stay the same and survive.

"Self" in Nursing

Finally, nursing's emphasis on the "therapeutic use of self" in effective nursing practice may actually make it harder for us to make our critiques of important issues confronting the profession more objective. We're taught that one of our greatest tools is bringing our "self" to the interactions with patients and families in ways that are healing. Nursing is emotional work. We're with people during highly emotional times, whether difficult or joyous. We're with patients and their families when death is near, during serious illness, at births, when they have to toilet, and when they're in pain. A recent commentary by Thomas Schwarz pointed out that some of these experiences can lead to secondary post-traumatic stress, burnout, and walking away from a job.[5] When we're operating on a complex and sometimes overwhelming emotional level, it may be difficult to transcend emotions in our arguments on issues. So it's not surprising that some nurses are unable to set aside their anger or distress when writing a letter to the editor about an issue and even to turn such emotions into an attack on the person expressing a position on an issue, particularly when the issue touches the emotional context of the letter writer's experience. It may take an expert level of practice to master the art of removing the "self" from intellectual discussions of issues when the emotional context of the issue needs to take a backseat. Moreover, if nursing is seen as being all about "self," then someone who critiques the status quo may be guilty not of an intellectual failing but of a personal one. This would, of course, lead to attacks not on the issue at hand but on the self that voices what may be considered heretical opinions.

It's encouraging to see nurses who feel proud of their profession. Many of us see it as one of the most important professions, because we serve people in their most troubling and vulnerable times, and we often work in abusive environments and for relatively little pay. No wonder nurses want to see themselves as angels and lash out at the messengers (such as Belcher) who find that analogy unnecessary and even troubling. Without that, what would be left to keep us in this work? How many nurses hold on to this image out of fear that losing it will leave them without a raison d'être? Can nursing survive without open discussion and debate on the critical issues of our times?

These questions demand that nurses be prepared for open, honest dialogue about the important issues confronting the profession. While the annual Gallup poll on the public's ratings of the ethics of various professions continues to rank nursing as the most trusted, that trust may be misplaced if nurses cannot demonstrate the courage to challenge the traditions in nursing and health care in ways that are reasoned, articulate, and respectful of those who disagree. The profession's future and the health of the public depend on nurses' courage and skill in challenging the status quo.

4

Moral Integrity and Regret in Nursing

Lydia L. Moland

Nursing literature is rife with stories of conflict. Nurses describe themselves in perpetual struggles with physicians, with hospital managers, with uncooperative patients and demanding families. They recount repeated battles over the allocation of insurance funds and over administration of the ever-shrinking resources of managed care. Many describe themselves as deeply dissatisfied with the current health care system, with nurses leaving the profession in alarming numbers because of this dissatisfaction. Conflict in the workplace is certainly not unique to nursing; every occupation has its characteristic tensions and potential for exhaustion and disillusionment. But behind nursing's description of its specific trials lurks a more disturbing claim, namely that nurses are consistently unable to maintain their integrity in their work. Some writers on nursing in fact claim that the conflicts that make integrity elusive for nurses are systemic, built into the occupation itself. Nursing's typical conflicts, in other words, cannot be explained away by the particulars of a dishonest boss, incompetent management, or dysfunctional coworkers. They are generated specifically by what the role of a nurse entails. Nurses often describe these conflicts as moral dilemmas that they feel powerless to resolve in an ethically satisfactory way. They are left with lingering regret no matter which of the

I thank those who have shared their experiences in nursing and expertise on the nursing crisis, especially Perri Strawn, and also Suzanne Gordon, Sylvain Trepannier, Aliina Hirschoff, Suzanne Smith, Peter Schwartz, and Bret Doyle. Thanks also to Bernard Prusak and the members of MIT's Workshop on Gender and Philosophy for their comments on earlier drafts of the chapter.

dilemma's options they pursue. They trace their powerlessness to the nature of nursing itself.

This charge is cause for serious reflection. Certainly it is of concern for the health care industry: if nurses cannot maintain their integrity in their work, we have reason to fear for our health. Indeed, if current trends continue, the ratio of nurses to those in need of care will decrease by 40 percent in the first decades of this century.[1] But beyond pragmatic concerns, the idea of an occupation that consistently prevents its participants from acting with integrity presents a deeper philosophical and ethical challenge. What would it mean to say that it is impossible for members of a certain occupation to preserve their integrity? What happens to agents who experience a systematic loss of integrity? Why might nurses be especially vulnerable to such loss? If this special vulnerability exists, what is to be done about it?

I begin, in the first part, by sketching a preliminary definition of integrity and linking it to an agent's self-understanding. I then attempt to isolate exactly what makes it difficult for nurses to feel that they act with integrity. In the second part, I evaluate the regret that accompanies a nurse's inability to do what she thinks is right.[2] I ask what role that regret plays in the assessment of a nurse's actions and what the regret itself indicates about her integrity. I conclude that in the current system of health care and because of the complex range of tasks nurses undertake, regret is unfortunately sometimes an unavoidable component of nurses' integrity. In fact, when the wish to avoid the discomforts of regret becomes too strong, nurses are sometimes led to act in ways that diminish their integrity even as they attempt to preserve it.

My intent is not to propose specific solutions to the current nursing shortage. Neither is it to espouse a particular ethical theory and then apply it to the nursing profession. I rather suggest that the example of nursing highlights the limitations of certain theoretical assumptions about integrity and regret, and that it focuses our attention on other necessary aspects of integrity, such as choosing principles appropriate to one's commitments. Examining nursing's struggles also encourages us to study the vocabulary nurses use to describe their work, specifically prominent concepts such as caring and advocacy. It encourages us to ask what is meant by these very laden terms and whether they are being interpreted in a way that makes it more difficult for nurses to feel that they act with integrity. Examining nursing through the lens of integrity can both enhance our sensitivity to these challenges in nursing and, more broadly, to the complexities of particular ethical experience.

Integrity and Self-Understanding

Integrity is often defined as the correlation between actions on the one hand and beliefs, principles, or convictions on the other.[3] If an agent believes that stealing is wrong, acting with integrity requires her not to steal. A person claiming an unwavering commitment to family who then abandons her parents in their old age is not acting with integrity. Although there are qualities that every agent must possess in order to act with integrity, integrity is in an important sense a deeply personal phenomenon.[4] The standards of personal integrity vary widely: one's integrity can consist of being a faithful and supportive friend, of adhering to certain dietary restrictions, or of sustaining specific standards in one's business relations.

Integrity also requires a correlation between our self-understanding and actions. If I understand myself to be a teacher, that understanding informs the way that I treat students. It will influence my attitude toward others in my profession and my sense of my function in the community. My identity, who I understand myself to be, gives me reasons for actions. My description of myself—and my acting in accordance with this description—gives my life coherence and purpose.[5]

Who I believe myself to be and what I believe I should do are thus often connected in a relatively straightforward way. This is certainly true of many professional or vocational identities. Being a pharmacist gives an agent an obligation and a reason to dispense medications conscientiously, a musician has reason to rehearse, a journalist has reason to investigate and report, and so forth. When a person acts according to the norms of her identity, there is a consistency between her self-understanding and her actions. Acting according to one's self-understanding, in other words, is one source of integrity.

Of course life does not always leave the way clear for us to act with integrity. Difficult decisions can leave us choosing between two evils, feeling that neither option allows us to act according to our principles or our self-understanding. As the workplace is typically an environment in which compromise is required, it provides ample opportunity for such conflict. In addition to making necessary compromises, employees can easily find themselves subordinate to those whose ethical beliefs they do not share. They may then be asked to act in ways they consider unethical. A police officer may be called on to lie and so violate her belief that lying is wrong; an accountant may be asked to misrepresent company profits; a teacher might be required to follow a curriculum that she finds ineffective or counterproductive. Because integrity is deeply linked to our personal projects and our ability to do what we believe is right, being prevented from acting with integrity can be the source of great psychological distress. Not being able to live up to her self-understanding weakens the agent's sense of self-value. Being repeatedly prevented from fulfilling an obligation within a role erodes an agent's integrity and with it her self-esteem.

Nurses claim that their integrity is under attack from two directions. First, they are frequently unable to do what they think is right for a patient. Second, they are routinely prevented from living up to their self-understanding as nurses. This second claim requires a closer look at what nurses' self-understanding is and how it is formed. For centuries, nursing has been promoted as a calling, an altruistic expression of selfless care and compassion.[6] It has been identified with traditionally female and specifically maternal virtues such as sympathy, nurturing, and long-suffering. That these virtues still survive as standards is obvious in the profession's continued veneration of an idealized Florence Nightingale.[7] Even where there is no mention of this patron saint of nursing, the rhetoric of care, of changing people's lives, helping those who suffer, and being compassionate is a dominant theme in nurses' description of their work. In a major campaign aiming to address the nursing shortage, Johnson & Johnson has posted personal statements from a wide range of nurses, many of which support this interpretation. The theme of this campaign is "Dare to Care."[8]

Not surprisingly, nursing draws people who are attracted by difficult and sometimes unrewarding labor, who find fulfillment in helping others. When described primarily as "caring," nursing appeals to people who understand themselves to be empathetic, compassionate, and patient. It requires devoting one's life to a task that will, under current circumstances, demand much and perhaps return little in the way of gratitude or compensation. Because of this combination of factors, it is not unusual to find articulations of nursing such as the following: "The end or purpose of nursing is the well-being of other people. This end is not a scientific end; it is a moral end. . . . The wise and humane application of knowledge and skill comprises the art of nursing. *Therefore, nursing is a moral art*."[9] For people drawn to this ideal, nursing is no ordinary profession but a calling, a response to a greater cause. This moral status of nursing is prominent in many nurses' self-understanding and sense of self-worth.[10]

Portraying nursing as a moral art exposes nurses to unique and sometimes painful pressures. As an example, it vilifies some motives for doing one's job and sanctifies others. Consider a nurse who, in 1888, wrote anonymously to *Trained Nurse*, signing her name "Candor":

> Where there is one nurse with a missionary spirit . . . there are forty-nine others who are obliged to make the humiliating confession: "I am a nurse

because I must earn a living for myself and those dependent on me, because my nursing is well-paid, honorable, and to me interesting."

The fact that "Candor" describes this "confession" as "humiliating" is striking. There are few other professions in which the acknowledgement that one undertook the work because it was respectable, interesting, and supported a family would be humiliating. Yet "Candor" describes a culture in which it is shameful to become a nurse for reasons that are not expressly altruistic. "Candor," however, refuses to accept this shame:

> Of course this spirit of self-immolation is very beautiful and lovely, but is it practical? Is it the motive power which had induced the army of sensible, practical women to take up this work? Let us be honest, even at the sacrifice of sentiment. Let us not hesitate to do a good deed when opportunity offers, but let us not try to make people believe we are angels and that to do good is the chief object in our lives, with a small remuneration thrown in, to which we scarcely give a thought.[11]

That "Candor" was going against the grain by suggesting this more practical approach is clear from nursing literature of the time. More surprisingly, contemporary literature confirms that, now as then, nurses often describe their work in terms of self-sacrifice and altruism rather than in practical terms of competence, expertise, and financial stability. The pride in being chosen for this mission increases nurses' identification with their occupation. It is not "just a job." It is a calling that reflects the individual's moral merit.

A nurse's identification with her vocation is also intensified by her daily dealings with life-and-death situations and with matters concerning human dignity and autonomy. Nurses are entrusted with the lives and physical well-being of strangers. Should they neglect any aspect of their job, the consequences may well be life threatening. Nurses have immediate access to confidential information about their patients and often see them in humiliating and vulnerable situations. For these reasons, nurses have, we hope, an especially intense sense of responsibility and professional integrity.[12] They justifiably take pride in their ability to negotiate these delicate and volatile situations.

These factors—the traditional description of nurses as embodying empathetic virtues, the idea that nursing is a moral profession, and the gravity of its subject matter—potentially strengthen the nurse's identification with her occupation.[13] Like all agents, she acts on a description of herself that gives her life coherence and meaning. But this coherence is under additional moral pressures that few professions share. While some other professions do deal directly with life and death, most do not rely on their members' altruistic, self-sacrificing, and compassionate natures. Nurses are told that they are uniquely suited to a very demanding task, and that sense often creates increased identification with their profession. Such close identification with one's occupation could, in an ideal world, be a source of moral strength and purpose. Nurses could feel themselves fortified for the difficult task at hand by referring to the nature of their calling.

The reality, however, is that this strong identification becomes a source of tension under the stressful realities of hospital care.[14] The most obvious starting point for understanding this is to examine the physician-nurse relationship. Both physicians and nurses deal regularly with life and death issues; both are members of an occupation with a long and venerated history. Clearly, their interactions are meant to be cooperative and productive, with each contributing an essential part to the joint project of health. Nevertheless, the physician-nurse relationship is often fraught with tension. Nursing literature recounts persistent conflict and sometimes open hostility between doctors and nurses.[15] Although the immediate causes of these conflicts vary, the root of the problem is often attributed to job descriptions that are then portrayed as mutually exclusive: nurses, as it is sometimes put, are concerned with care, while physicians are concerned with cure.

We can trace this simplistic dichotomization of two obviously complex jobs to the history and current practice of medicine. Nursing was and is a predominantly female profession, with female nurses originally expected to be obedient and unassertive assistants to male doctors. In the last century, nurses have consequently encountered all the traditional problems associated with women's bid for equality in the workplace. But nursing's case is made yet more intractable than the case of women in other professions because not only are the vast majority of nurses female, but the profession *itself* is built on what are still considered female virtues, including the sympathy, compassion, and nurturing described above. Although certain gains have been made against this tradition, the history of nurses as simple extensions of physicians' orders ("the physician's hand") is still clearly visible in hospital hierarchy.[16] Physicians are not required to consult nurses or take their opinions into account. A nurse, depending on her particular relationship to a doctor, can make recommendations, but she cannot make fundamental decisions about the kind of care the patient will receive. Except in cases of extreme physician negligence or incompetence, nurses are legally obligated to carry out the prescribed treatment even if they know it is against the patient's wishes or believe it is not in the patient's best interest.

For these reasons, some have argued that nursing is a subordinate occupation and, because it lacks autonomy and flexibility, does not even qualify as a profession.[17]

True to the history of nursing as a feminine and moral art, the care that nurses provide is often described solely as emotional, compassionate support. Its archetypal image is the nurse comforting a suffering patient, providing sympathy and emotional comfort in an otherwise technical, inhuman world. Without a doubt, the personal attention nurses routinely provide to patients is crucial to the healing process. But when described exclusively in these emotional terms, it risks not being respected by a traditionally male and increasingly technical profession. Nurses struggle to find a place for their observations of a patient's emotional and mental well-being in medicine's analysis of the patient's physical well-being. When this language of emotion and sympathy is not heard, neither are nurses. Caring, in other words, is not a powerful position from which to bargain: this is especially true since physicians can claim to have technology, science, objectivity, and progress on their side. Additionally, if nurses depict themselves as responding to a higher moral calling, they are likely to be taken advantage of by those who view their own occupations more pragmatically. It will be easier to pay nurses less, consult them less, and ignore their low levels of job satisfaction if it is believed that what is truly satisfying about the job is its opportunities for selfless altruism. The care vs. cure distinction, it seems, puts nurses at a distinct disadvantage, leaving them open to exploitation.

But what is meant here by care? What is it that nurses do that is opposed to what physicians do? Caring, in everyday life, can mean many things: we can care for, that, and about things; we can also take care, and take care of something or someone.[18] Sometimes expertise and discipline are required in order to take care of something. Other times, caring entails emotional support and nurturing. Often, care requires both: it requires a competent assessment of what needs to be done, the knowledge of how to do it, and the sympathy to want to do it. But all too frequently, caring in nursing is described exclusively in emotional terms. It is then depicted as being in direct opposition to the physician's technical, science-based approach.

When treated as essentially synonymous with compassion and nurturing, the label "caring" underrepresents what nurses actually do. Part of caring, for instance, is being a patient advocate: as the etymology would suggest, speaking for that patient, promoting his wishes when he lacks the education, power, or strength to do so. Being such an advocate clearly requires the empathy necessary to hear and understand the patient's desires. But it also requires extensive knowledge of illnesses, medication, and possible treatments. It also requires the ability to communicate a patient's wishes to physicians in ways physicians understand. It may demand that the nurse argue, agitate, and fight for the patient against the doctor. This technical and even combative side of nursing is often overlooked in both the public's representation of nurses and nurses' representation of themselves.

Clearly both caring and patient advocacy are needed to ensure a patient's recovery. Yet because caring is construed as the essence of nursing and then defined with little reference to the technical competence nurses have, nurses claim that their attempts at patient advocacy often go unheeded.

Certainly we want to preserve the presence of caring in the recovery process, and there are aspects of caring that require nonquantifiable, nontechnical qualities such as empathy, compassion, and intuition. But restricting nursing to *this* aspect of caring while neglecting other equally essential aspects puts *both* aspects in danger of being ignored.

It is worth considering how this emotion-based definition of caring makes it difficult for nurses to feel that they act with integrity. Perhaps the most commonly cited conflict in the nursing literature concerns patients who express a desire to die but whose doctors nevertheless continue to prescribe treatment.[19] Here, nurses complain, doctors tend to give priority to treating the disease over respecting the patient's autonomy. This prioritization, they further claim, is supported by a health care system that favors technological solutions and sees death as a failure.[20] Nurses, whose closer contact with the patient often enables them to learn more about the patient's wishes, are often left feeling that the patient should have been allowed to die. Clearly every case is different, and often physicians have good reasons for their decisions. But nurses describe feeling that, because physicians are not required to take nurses' perspectives into account, care for patients as persons—rather than as opportunities for experimentation or professional success—is disregarded. And, to repeat, nurses are the ones left administering the treatment, prescribed by the doctor, that prevents the patient's death. Nurses who are caught disobeying a doctor's orders to resuscitate risk serious professional and legal consequences. Other frequently cited conflicts include when a nurse is asked to be dishonest with a patient about his prognosis or the possible effects of treatment; when she is asked to administer treatments she finds unnecessary; and when she confronts a doctor's unwillingness to prescribe the level of pain medication that a patient, in the nurse's judgment, needs. In such cases, the nurse's attention to the patient's emotional state is disregarded and sometimes even seen as a hindrance to the treatment the physician prescribes. Again, the nurse's more personal connection with the patient makes her feel these conflicts as a threat to her self-understanding as a caring patient's advocate.

Because nursing is so often described as a moral art and a calling, nurses frequently characterize these disputes with physicians as *moral* disagreements rather than professional or clinical disagreements. Thus, when a nurse fails to convince the doctor of what she thinks is right, she experiences this as a moral failure. Not doing what we think is morally right can destroy our sense of internal harmony, our sense of wholeness: this we describe as a loss of integrity. And indeed, nurses frequently describe their inability to do what they believe is best for the patient as a loss of integrity.[21]

Ironically, a nurse's job is difficult for her in large part when she is good at what she does. If she did not care about her patients, she would not experience her powerlessness to do what she believes is best for them so keenly. The more strongly a nurse feels that attending to the patient's needs is part of her self-understanding, the more likely she will be to intervene on a patient's behalf, to find herself in conflict with physicians, and to be unable to act on her moral judgment. If she did not feel that her empathetic nature was an important part of her identity, being unable to help the suffering patient would not be so painful a source of distress. If she did not believe her occupation was inherently moral, she would not feel her moral integrity to be so threatened and, consequently, would not feel a threat to her sense of self.[22]

The consequences to a nurse's sense of self in conflicted situations can be devastating. Adele Waring Pike, a nurse writing about nurses, recounts her experience as a novice nurse and the disillusionment and moral suffering it caused her:

> It never occurred to me . . . that I would have cause to doubt my ability to maintain my moral integrity. My confidence in my ability to maintain my moral integrity was quickly shattered early in my career, however, as I encountered moral conflicts I had never imagined. . . . My struggle to find firm moral ground was complicated by conflicts with powerful physicians and administrators over how patients were to be cared for at the end of life, how pain and suffering were to be managed, over staff competence, over my right to participate in decisions that I was expected to implement. I often experienced moral distress over my inability to act in accordance with what I thought to be right and good and helpful.[23]

Pike's quote is doubly instructive. First, she indicates that she had never imagined that working as a nurse could threaten her moral integrity. This, it seems to me, is further evidence of the unique situation of nursing. In what other profession would one expect no occasion for moral compromise? If the goals of nursing are thought to be so pure that nurses are not trained to expect tension and the need for compromise, it is no wonder that nurses feel shocked and disillusioned when faced with the realities of hospital work. Secondly, we see again that these perceived "failures"—failures for which she was not prepared and that she did not expect—are described as moral failures: as an inability to do what was "right or good or helpful." It is no wonder, given this lack of preparation, intense identification with the profession, and persistent tension in nursing practice, that nurses describe acute psychological distress.

This ongoing conflict suggests a greater tension within the role of nursing itself. Clearly part of a nurse's duty is to follow the orders of a doctor; when this duty regularly conflicts with her obligations as a patient advocate, the problem seems intractable. This is particularly true if the nurse is not prepared for or given the tools to handle the conflict. The nurse is left with a dilemma: she either acts against her sense of herself as a nurse or risks losing her job. If nursing continues to recruit those who see caring as part of their ethical identity, new nurses will be likely to experience the same disillusionment and distress. If nursing education and literature continue to describe nurses' work primarily in terms of caring and self-sacrifice, the disillusionment is likely to worsen. And as long as nursing is understood as a primarily ethical undertaking, nurses will continue to experience these failures in a way that threatens their fundamental sense of self. It is not difficult to imagine that a job that does not allow an agent to preserve her integrity because she is good at what she does can lead to acute job dissatisfaction. Although certainly not the only factor in the nursing shortage, the especially personal nature of this moral distress undoubtedly contributes to it.

Integrity and Regret

I began with the question of whether nursing's plight is distinctive and have answered in the affirmative. Nursing's basis in caring—and the persistent focus on a certain limited definition of caring—both makes it more important to a nurse's moral sense of self that she act as she thinks best and makes it more difficult. The dichotomy between caring and curing encourages the impression that nurses' work is opposed to physicians' work, so intensifying conflict between the two. Nursing's daily dealings with life-and-death issues exacerbate this already fraught situation. Hierarchical hospital structure combined with nursing's history and predominantly female membership burden the profession with the problems both of subordinate labor groups and of women in the workplace. Clearly many nurses suffer persistent moral distress related to issues of integrity and self-understanding. Given this particularly charged situation, what possible relief might there be?

An obvious solution to this problem is the "professionalization" of nursing: that is, changing nurses' self-understanding by emphasizing their technical skills and medical expertise and de-emphasizing their nurturing role. Such a change—already to some extent attempted—seems to have the potential to relieve nurses' moral distress in that their self-understanding would be based on impersonal, technical expertise rather than the intricacies of a patient's needs and wishes. A revised self-understanding would also be less likely to put the nurse at odds with doctors. The professionalization movement also trains nurses to do more traditionally medical work—such as the work of nurse-practitioners or anesthesiologists—and so allows them to gain status and some autonomy. Other demands made by the professionalization movement—for higher pay, better benefits, and more flexible schedules—combat the impression that nurses' work is based in self-sacrifice and so requires no reward. Some claim that these developments have indeed improved nursing conditions.[24]

It is indicative of the centrality of the emotional, nonquantifiable aspect of caring to nurses' self-understanding, however, that the professionalization movement has met with considerable internal resistance. A significant number of nurses seem to fear that, should caring be de-emphasized, nursing will lose its essence. Ann Bradshaw, for example, defends the need for nurses' traditional caring in the promotion of health: "Comforting, chatting with, holding hands with, feeding, washing, bathing, cleaning other people when they are sick, were all traditional nursing tasks, and in many circumstances essential for patient care. This is no less true at the end of the twentieth century."[25] Soma Hewa and Robert Hetherington argue that the bid for professionalization actually backfires since those who go into nursing do not find job satisfaction in professional, technical expertise. The "growing pressures to implement a mechanistic medical model in nursing," they write, "tend to undermine such basic values of the nursing profession and lead to job dissatisfaction, stress, frustration and confrontation between nurses, physicians and health care administrators."[26] Maslach claims that burnout increases when nurses begin to think of themselves as technicians rather than caregivers.[27] Studies have also shown that increasing pay only temporarily relieves a nurse's exhaustion and disillusionment with her job.[28] Replacing the centrality of caring with a less fraught self-understanding and an increase in resources proves, interestingly, not to be enough. Despite the fact that a "professionalized" self-conception might alleviate the moral distress so prevalent in hospital settings, nurses are reluctant to adopt this new conception because it threatens to leave a crucial component of nursing's self-conception behind.

Nor have nurses reacted positively to the suggestion that their description of moral dilemmas simply reflects an incorrect ordering of moral principles. Some nurses resist the idea that if they would only adopt principles such as those put forward in the medical ethics literature—principles of autonomy, beneficence, justice, and so forth—their ethical dilemmas would disappear. Some nurses have argued that the challenges that nurses face are in fact fundamentally different from those that physicians face and that the same principles cannot apply to both.[29] Nurses have also shown themselves to be skeptical of autonomy- or rights-based approaches to ethics: Susan Reverby reports for instance that "nurses have often rejected liberal feminism . . . because of some deep understandings of the limited promise of equality and autonomy in a health-care system they see as flawed and harmful. In an often inchoate way, such nurses recognize that those who claim the autonomy of rights often run the risk of rejecting altruism and caring itself."[30] Others have suggested that the idea of fixed principles is inappropriate in a vocation as clearly based in the variability of the human condition as nursing is, concluding that "the assumption that ethical theory is sufficient to cope with suffering is simply wrong."[31] One need not agree with these claims to recognize that many nurses see the conflicts they experience as resisting easy analysis and resolution. Again, what is striking is that nurses seem unwilling to relinquish the distress they feel; they hold to the uniqueness of their predicament against theoretical analysis. Are nurses doomed to diminished integrity because their self-understanding consistently presents them with conflicting obligations?

Moral philosophers have long grappled with the question of whether it is possible for an agent to have two conflicting obligations: to have, that is, a real moral dilemma. For our purposes, I think Ruth Barcan Marcus's assessment of moral dilemmas is instructive. In "Moral Dilemmas and Consistency," Marcus discusses various philosophical positions (she specifically discusses formalism and intuitionism) that suggest that there are no real moral dilemmas, only misunderstandings of principles and their hierarchy.[32] These misunderstandings lead the agent to believe that there is no ethically satisfactory solution to the situation in question. The fear that there is no solution then produces moral distress, which is expressed as guilt, remorse, regret, shame, self-reproach, and so forth.[33] Marcus proceeds to criticize this dismissive analysis of moral dilemmas. Claiming that moral dilemmas do not actually exist, Marcus argues, implies that the guilt or regret that results from the agony of a perceived dilemma is also misguided. Because these negative emotions have no real cause, they can only be considered sentimental or pathological. According to Marcus, however, this assessment is "false to the facts . . . It is inadequate to insist that feelings of guilt about the rejected alternative are mistaken and that assumption of guilt is inappropriate." Dilemmas, she instead claims, are themselves "data of a kind." Specifically, they are data that need "to be taken into account in the future conduct of our lives. If we are to avoid dilemmas we must be motivated to do so."[34] In other words, the distress produced when an agent confronts a dilemma provides a critical motivation to change the circumstances that give rise to the difficulty: "To deny the appropriateness or correctness of ascriptions of guilt is to weaken the impulse to make such arrangements."[35] The distress motivates the agent to seek the origin of the dilemma and to alter the situation so as to avoid a similar clash in the future. For this reason, the distress of dilemmas should not be explained away.

Clearly, the guilt or regret nurses experience when unable to resolve a dilemma point to much that is inadequate in the health care system. As Marcus's theory would suggest, these painful responses sometimes motivate nurses to pursue reforms that would eliminate that regret. I think further that nurses would welcome support from Marcus for their claim that the dilemmas of hospital life are not simply the result of misordered principles. Yet it seems that a further observation is in order: while moral distress can sometimes assist us in motivating change that genuinely solves the problem and so makes continued regret unnecessary, eliminating distress itself unfortunately does not necessarily mean that the problem has been solved. Moral distress can just as easily be eliminated by evading the problem as by effecting a solution. If nursing is defined as caring as opposed to physicians' curing, it can seem that the only way out is to disregard the complexity of the problem: to care and, in so doing, to oppose the physician, or to cure by being simply an assistant to the physician.

That this is a real possibility is made clear through Adele Waring Pike's research on the role of regret in what she calls nurses' integrity-preserving practices. As part of this research, Pike identifies various nursing practices that *do* protect the agent from moral distress and its symptoms but in fact *do not* solve the problem. These practices, Pike subsequently argues, do not preserve the agent's integrity. I turn now to these cases and to the implicit aspects of integrity that, I believe, they make explicit. I think they further clarify the complex conception of care that is at the foundation of nursing's self-conception and necessary to nurses' pursuit of integrity.

Pike first discusses the case of a young nurse who eliminates regret by interpreting herself solely as the assistant to the doctor.[36] This nurse forbids herself to dwell on discrepancies between the patient's wishes or needs and the treatment a physician prescribes. She refuses to give a patient even aspirin without a doctor's permission. She may sympathize and commiserate with the patient, regretting with him his discomfort and distress. But so long as she believes she can do nothing about it, she feels no real ambivalence about the patient's pain.

If this nurse persists in seeing her job only as following the doctor's orders, she will not recognize complex situations in which a patient's needs and a doctor's orders conflict. She is thus less likely to experience dilemmas and the regret that they create. Instead, she preserves her sense of integrity by acting consistently under a principle: the principle stipulating that she act exclusively on the orders of the doctor. She may justify this as care, claiming that she is caring for the patient both by commiserating with him and by following the doctor's orders.

Our initial definition of integrity, we will remember, was acting consistently according to one's principles and self-understanding. The above example necessitates two modifications of this original definition. The first is that consistency can in fact sometimes interfere with integrity. Surely we would not want to describe the nurse in the above example as acting with integrity, despite her faithful adherence to principle. Surely her refusal to take the patient's pain seriously detracts from the value we might attribute to her consistency. Holding steadfastly to a principle is not enough: a fact, I believe, explained by the second modification, namely that beyond requiring that we act consistently on any principle, integrity requires us to act according to an *appropriate* self-understanding. It seems clear that this nurse is abandoning a pivotal part of the self-understanding necessary to be a nurse, namely caring as actual patient advocacy. If a nurse's self-understanding does not include this central component of nursing, it is surely incorrect to describe her as acting with integrity. If the description of nursing's goals as I have sketched them is accurate, this nurse is not pursuing, much less achieving, the goals nursing is committed to pursuing. Nursing requires attention both to doctor and to patient and, in this case, the nurse is ignoring the patient. The absence of regret, a result of her consistently acting on principle, does not in this case result in integrity. Nor does it indicate that the nurse, motivated by her regret, has solved the dilemma at hand. She has, we could perhaps say, instead *dis*solved the dilemma—made it go away in a manner no less dismissive than the formalists' or intuitionists' reduction of dilemmas to a misapplication of principles. Her overreliance on principle, her inadequate self-understanding, and her oversimplified understanding of the work itself interfere with her ability to act with integrity.

Pike also documents nurses who ignore the complexity of the situation by going to the other extreme: by routinely disobeying doctors in order to do what they believe is in the patient's interest. For example, a nurse may clandestinely administer drugs that are not prescribed, allow a patient to die despite a doctor's orders to resuscitate, or undermine a patient's confidence in the doctor. She may make this behavior habitual, allowing her contempt for what she perceives to be doctors' skewed priorities to dictate ever more decisions. This may result in the complete disintegration of the mission she shares with doctors. She, too, may justify this to herself as care, as putting the patient first regardless of the unfeeling doctor.

Such actions threaten integrity, Pike claims, not because they are clandestine, but because when made habitual, they can diminish the nurse's capacity to feel regret when a situation calls for it. They can allow the nurse to act as if she is above the fray, superior to what she sees to be mindless obedience. According to Pike, such moral self-exculpation threatens a nurse's integrity even more than does her inability to help a patient in the way she thinks best. This is true despite the fact that nurses who habitually disobey doctors *do* act consistently and under a principle: they do "not exhibit an insincerity of moral purpose or lack of substantive moral commitments. On the contrary they [are] very clear about the values they cherish . . . and deeply committed to them."[37] Yet they "express . . . pride in their [resistance] practice, rather than regret over not having been able to take action that would have affected a better patient outcome."[38] Integrity-diminishing practices—as Pike calls them—do not have "what else could I have done" responses.[39] This moral callousness will threaten as long as nurses are both encouraged to see themselves as carers as opposed to curers and then put in a hierarchy that prevents them from caring in a meaningful way.

In other words, such resistance practices may serve the immediate need of allowing the nurse to feel she is acting in accordance with principles of patient advocacy. When made habitual, these actions can be carried out without regret and so dispel the consciousness of the dilemma that called for resistance to begin with. In the end, such nurses except themselves from having to reckon with moral dilemmas—a "solution" that, far from eliminating these dilemmas, may lead the nurse to act as if moral quandaries were artificial and thus not to be taken seriously. Like the nurse who acts only on the doctor's orders and so does not engage in the full difficulty of the situation, the renegade nurse denies the reality of the dilemma, taking refuge in consistency. Also like the unthinkingly obedient nurse, the consistently disobedient nurse chooses to ignore a central part of nursing's conception, namely its role alongside doctors in the cooperative project of health care. When a nurse's disobedience extends to this kind of subversion, she also ceases to be an advocate in the sense of being someone who gives voice to and pleads the case of someone else. She is no longer the patient's voice to the doctor; she is instead obstructing the relationship and perhaps threatening the patient's recovery. Care cannot be *this* easy, either, since competent hospital care requires communication and cooperation with doctors. But if caring is defined as directly opposed to the doctor's project of curing, it can seem that the only way for the nurse to do her job is to defy the doctor in whatever ways she can.

Two essential aspects of integrity are, to repeat, emphasized by the case of nursing. The first is the limited value of consistency. Part of integrity is not valuing consistency and mental comfort over an honest evaluation of an ethically problematic situation. Certainly increased or sustained attention to these difficult situations is likely to make a nurse continue to think she lacks exactly what she is seeking, namely integrity. One experienced nurse in Pike's survey, for instance, recounts the varying and sometimes inconsistent practices she uses to cope with dilemmas. Because of this inconsistency, the nurse concludes, "I don't know how ethical I am."[40] But Pike claims—plausibly, it seems to me—that we should evaluate the integrity of actions not only in terms of consistency, but in terms of appropriate deliberation and compromise.[41] She writes of this self-doubting nurse: "Edna alternated between practices that diminished her integrity and those that preserved it as she struggled to act in accordance with her cherished values and negotiate relations of power in health care organizations. The inconsistency in her practices is what led her to question her moral integrity." But Pike concludes that Edna acts as ethically as possible and with as much integrity as possible. What is essential to this integrity is Edna's willingness to struggle, to realize that every case will be different and many will present dilemmas. Edna acts with integrity that confronts the full meaning of caring, caring in all its complexity, tension, and necessary compromise. She neither clings to a principle that prevents her from engaging with the difficulty of the situation nor abandons a central part of her self-understanding as a nurse in order to simplify her work. Important to note here is that Edna does sometimes do things that relieve her distress: a definition of integrity cannot require an agent to struggle without end. But she tempers these distress-relieving practices with practices that engage with the full difficulty of being a nurse.

Another way to view this necessary tension is to say that Edna is engaging with a fuller, more complex definition of caring than are the other two nurses. The first nurse understands care, insofar as she understands it at all, as submitting to the authority of the doctor. She has shut out completely the emotional, supportive, empathetic aspect of care. Nurses who act against doctors on principle act on another inadequate, oversimplified definition of care. They understand it to be ministering to the patient's desires regardless of the doctor's opinions. In fact, caring requires a combination of these and other attitudes. This complexity, again, is unlikely to make the nurse feel she is acting consistently since vastly different and seemingly conflicting actions are often expected of her. But choosing a path that enables her to act consistently at the cost of confronting the full complexity of her job is not a satisfactory solution—for her sense of integrity or for the patient's health.

This leads us to the second essential aspect of integrity that nursing highlights, namely the importance of ascertaining whether the self-understanding on which an agent acts is appropriate. In order to act with integrity, nurses must adopt principles that further the profession's goals: promotion of health through advocating and caring for patients on the one hand and assisting doctors in patients' treatments on the other. Nurses who ignore one or another of these goals—either by following doctors' orders unquestioningly or not at all—are, again, not fulfilling the ideals of nursing and so not acting with integrity. But if these goals form the nurses' self-conception, she will tend to feel regret when it is, as Pike argues, necessary. Integrity in nursing requires rejecting the claim that care is unidimensional and simply opposed to cure. It requires seeing instead that caring some-times demands actions that are in tension with each other. It then involves feeling regret when those conflicting demands cannot be satisfactorily met.

But there is another sense in which this struggle and regret reinforce the definition of integrity as acting consistently, according to principles or self-understanding. Confronting an ethical dilemma with integrity requires the agent to maintain commitment to an ideal regardless of the difficulty of doing so. In the case of nurses, this ideal is the need for caring and advo-cacy in health care. A full understanding of these components of nursing's specific ideal is essential to being a good nurse. Yet typical hospital hierar-chy, as we have seen, makes providing this care very difficult. A nurse's willingness to struggle with the complexities of this faulty system and her willingness to feel regret when she is unable to do as she thinks best reflect her conviction that care is indeed essential to health care. These battles, in other words, are evidence of nurses' dedication to a complex description of caring despite sometimes being denied the satisfaction of acting according to that description. Integrity and regret are, in this case, not incompatible.

To claim that it is possible to act with integrity while being pre-vented from doing what one thinks is right is not in any way to belittle the distress nurses feel—it is not to say that in fact they are not experiencing a threat to integrity. They clearly are. This is especially true given many nurses' close identification with their role and the unique moral overtones commonly attributed to nursing. And if feeling regret in situations that allow of no satisfactory conclusion is part of maintaining moral integrity, nurses will continue to shoulder more than their fair share of regret.

But this overabundance of regret should not be equated any more than necessary with a loss of integrity. Nurses' integrity cannot be accounted for—at least in the current health care system—by adherence to principles without considering the specific challenges to integrity those principles present. I have claimed that the example of nursing forces us to modify the original definition of integrity in two ways. The first is that integrity cannot only be acting consistently. The examples of nurses who act consistently while disregarding essential aspects of care is evidence of this. The second is that integrity demands that a person act on an appropriate self-understanding. A nurse cannot act with integrity while disregarding the complex and sometimes conflicting demands of care. Attention to the complicated nature of caring is then part of the self-understanding indispensable to a nurse's integrity. Ideally, of course, nurses should be able to act on their commitments to care and patient advocacy without regret. But the persistence of this regret often indicates that nurses continue to struggle to fulfill the sometimes conflicting demands of patient care.

Perhaps some of this distress can be alleviated by increased awareness that acting on an appropriately complex concept of care presents nurses with a particularly difficult challenge. They cannot simply care and physicians simply cure, if by "caring" we mean only emotional support. Addressing nurses' experience of moral dilemmas and regret, then, requires that we temper the emotion-based definition of care with a more realistic presentation of what nurses actually do: the technical competencies they acquire, the high-level negotiations they undertake with physicians, the intricate assessments they must make in order to provide the care that is undoubtedly indispensable to health. It requires also that we are aware of nursing's history as a female profession and the struggles that this inheritance implies. If the public and physicians have this more realistic image of what nursing requires and what difficulties it faces, perhaps nurses will gain more of the respect and understanding they deserve.

Perhaps if our image of nursing is revised in this way, there will be fewer nurses who experience extreme disillusionment when their work presents conflicts they never imagined. If nurses themselves include a more complex image of care in their self-understanding, perhaps encountering the conflicts typical to nursing will not present so great a threat to nurses' sense of self. Perhaps more nurses will come to see the necessary compromises they make as an honest response to the complexity of caring and not as moral failure. Perhaps this will lessen the distress they suffer, allowing them to feel that they are acting with integrity even in persistent situations of compromise and regret.

5

Ethical Expertise and the Problem of the Good Nurse

Sioban Nelson

What is a good nurse? Is a good nurse necessarily a good person? These two questions, which stand at the interface between ethical reasoning and clinical judgment, are the subject of much discussion in nursing. In what follows, I will examine both the intellectual origins and contemporary manifestations of the trend to reframe expertise for practicing nurses as encompassing ethical competence. I will question the idea of a fundamental disposition toward the good as expressed by nursing scholars such as Patricia Benner, and argue that the equation of ethical and clinical expertise has alarming implications for nursing.

The "Home" of Ethics?

In his speech at Munich University, published in 1919 as "Politics as a Vocation," Max Weber raised the question, "Where is the natural ethical home of politics?"[1] It was a provocative question that Weber used to "open up" what he considered the habitually "closed" discussion of the political and ethical, where all participants simply declared themselves the moral superior of their opponents. With characteristic hardheadedness, Weber dismissed a reliance on a notion of "the good" as unhelpful in discussions about political ethics. He called instead for an appreciation of the plurality of ethical conduct that emerges from diverse contexts. He asked, "But is it

This chapter is an expansion of Sioban Nelson, "The Search for the Good in Nursing," *Nursing Philosophy* 5, no. 1 (2004).

true that any ethic of the world could establish commandments of identical content for erotic, business, familial, and official relations; for the relations to one's wife, to the green-grocer, the son, the competitor, the friend, the defendant?"[2] Weber was mounting an attack on what he termed the "Sermon on the Mount" posture of political ethics.[3] He took aim at the religious hypocrisy of both politicians and political analysts whose focus on the good, in Weber's view, masked the unmentionable fact that politics was essentially about power and that, as such, one would be wise to pay more attention to the deed than the discourse. In what follows I take up Weber's challenge to "tackle resolutely" the question of the natural home of ethics—in this case, nursing ethics.[4] To do so I examine the model of ethical expertise put forward by Patricia Benner in her later work on nursing expertise.[5] I question the religious and philosophical assumptions of this approach to both ethics and expertise, raise reservations about the utility and validity of narrative-based formulations of expertise—both ethical and clinical—and argue that blurring ethical and clinical competence blinds us to the political and structural constraints that define the parameters of nursing practice.

Expertise

Ask any nurse today about expertise in practice and the answer she or he provides will most likely be a tribute to the work of one woman. Quite simply, in her landmark 1984 work, *From Novice to Expert*, Patricia Benner changed the way nursing thinks about practice.[6] Benner developed a model for understanding nursing that both named and empowered the contextual decision making and clinical skill of those whom she considered to be "expert" nurses. She was strongly influenced by the feminist thinkers of the 1970s and 1980s, most particularly Carol Gilligan's notion of "women's ways of knowing."[7] Benner studied and worked with context-based thinkers in psychology and skill development who were mounting a strong critique of the contemporary robotics movement, eventually delineating the now famous five stages in skill acquisition: novice, advanced beginner, competent, proficient, and, finally, expert.[8]

The impact of this work was, and remains, remarkable. Benner's ideas radically resituated discussions of nursing practice, moving it from abstract theorization or simple skill checklists to the complex arena of contextualized learning and practice. Benner's model of the process through which nurses acquire skill and expertise led to the design of a major professional initiative, a clinical career pathway for nurses. In the effort to support the case that nurses should be rewarded at a level appropriate to their skill and performance, Benner delineated a widely accepted set of competencies that underpin her five stages of expertise.

For nursing this was more than an important text, it was a text that drilled down to and excavated the core of nursing practice, announced and articulated its importance to the world.[9] Twenty years later the star still shines on this work, and Benner has moved from the margins, critiquing abstract nursing theories, to a central place in nursing discourse where she is the world authority on the practice domain.

Benner's work has become the foundation of national competency frameworks adopted by professional associations and regulatory authorities in Canada, Australia, the United States, and elsewhere. It is the basis for a professional development and work organization model that has been widely adopted by hospitals and health providers.[10] The Benner model organizes care, nursing roles, career pathways, and salaries according to skill levels that correlate with the five-stage framework of novice to expert. Moreover, Benner has provided a wealth of writings for undergraduate and graduate nursing curricula throughout the world. The latest in a string of influential initiatives is the Carnegie-funded Study of Nursing Education.[11] In this capacity her work has defined, and continues to define, nursing practice and clinical expertise and explain how knowledge and skill are developed.

Benner argues that expertise is a function of a nurse's experience coupled with her accrued capacity to navigate complex clinical situations. According to Benner, as experts, nurses do not depend on mere "analytic principal rule (rule, guideline, maxim) to connect their understanding of the situation to an appropriate action."[12] From a deeply clinically and morally entrenched stance, Benner's expert nurse "has an intuitive grasp of the situation and zeroes in on the accurate region of the problem without wasteful consideration of a large range of unfruitful, alternative diagnoses and solutions."[13]

In her past research, which involved interviews, observation, and narrative development, Benner focused a much-needed lens on how nurses made clinical decisions. The task for nursing researchers, as part of this self-conscious project for the "articulation" of nursing practice, was to illuminate the clinical knowledge and skill that underpins excellence in nursing practice and to highlight the significance of this skill for patient care. The expert nurse was defined as someone whose outstanding clinical assessment skills, contextual knowledge, and experience come together so that he or she arrives at an intuitive grasp of the whole situation.

Narratives of Expertise

Fundamental to the development of Benner's model of expertise has been the production of practice narratives. When reading the compelling narratives produced by Benner's research over the past twenty years, one is impressed by the wonderfully skilled nurses, their clinical prowess, and their importance in managing patients, families, colleagues, and medicine to avert catastrophe. For hardworking and generally unappreciated nurses the narratives offer recognition and a powerful and empowering reframing of their role. However, in witnessing and applauding this reframing of practice some of its problematic aspects have been overlooked. First, the stories, which are carefully fashioned first-person accounts, are not neutral depictions of clinical practice. They were elicited by researchers who spent a great deal of time coaching their respondents about the precise narratives they were seeking. As such they do not reflect or reveal essential truths about all of nursing practice but create a very particular story about practice. This is a very important distinction. The narratives were developed collaboratively between the research team and the participants in a highly structured process.

In the first step, the preparation phase, nurses were made familiar with the nature of the interview process. Three weeks before being interviewed, they were asked to produce written stories of care with particular patients.

In the second step, setting the stage, nurses were "warmed up" and coached to create the desired interview milieu—one of everyday language in which they would feel comfortable relating their stories of practice. Coaching involved assisting participants in developing the desired tone and practice content. This took place in small groups, with group participation modeled by examples from the research team. Then, by listening to one another's narratives (within the group) each participant was encouraged to develop "salient" aspects of their own story over the course of three interviews. In this way future research participants practiced and were made comfortable relating their stories in first-person experiential terms.

In the third step, data collection, nurse participants took turns telling their narratives of patient care in their small groups. While they were relating their stories, the interviewer retraced the story and filled in the particulars about circumstances that arose in these narratives with respect to the nurse's major concerns. To address identified gaps in the narratives, the interviewers employed data collection guidelines consisting of probes that related to Benner's nine dimensions of expertise.

Typical probes included (a) What are all the hunches you have about this patient and what is wrong with him/her, based on what you know about him/her? (b) What do you think your hunch is based on? (c) Do you have any physical or emotional sensations associated with your hunch? Please describe; (d) How certain do you feel about this hunch?[14]

According to Benner, "by the second and third interview, nurses were well-versed on what we were seeking," and the desired narratives flowed "once the nurses became versed in their storytelling."[15]

Of particular interest to this discussion is the way in which narratives have been used to not only articulate clinical skill but to illustrate the idea of "the good" in nursing. "Narratives exemplify positive notions about what is good and not just the problems or deficits, and this is so whether or not the person can state formally or explicitly the notions of good that are being exemplified."[16]

It is this idea of the good, and expertise in relation to it, that I will now explore.

The Idea of the Good in Practice

To understand the idea of an essential good in practice it is necessary to briefly discuss the philosophical and methodological orientation of Benner's work. The philosophical approach that underpinned this landmark research combined a phenomenological understanding of being with a far older Aristotelian perspective on skill and virtue. The great contemporary representatives of Aristotelian ideas (also known as neo-Thomist after St. Thomas Aquinas) are the U.S. philosopher Alisdair MacIntyre and the Canadian, Charles Taylor.

MacIntyre is the famed author of *After Virtue* and an authority on Aristotle.[17] Charles Taylor is a well-known neo-Aristotelian philosopher whose life-long work represents a call for communitarian and humanist values and a sense of social connectedness as essential features of a civilized society. It is Taylor's conviction that human beings rely on openness to the divine source of affirmation in order to accede to their moral subjectivity. Taylor claims that the direct apprehensions of the needs of another or the intuited sense of the requirements of a principle are key elements of moral subjectivity. Critically for Taylor, this awareness of the good arises from the idea of a prereflective moral life shaping moral experience and motivating moral action.[18] Moral life is understood by Taylor as implicit rather than based on conscious awareness.[19]

As Benner has continued her research and writing in the area of expertise over the decades, the mark of Charles Taylor has become increasingly evident in her work. In Benner's words, "Charles Taylor's work provides the vision and example for examining notions of the good embedded in narratives and observations of actual practice."[20] Taylor returns the compliment, describing her work in nursing as providing "a paradigm area where Aristotle's model of judgment by phronesis is at home."[21]

The clearest indication of this Taylorian turn is the emergence in Benner's work of the idea that clinical expertise and moral status are one and the same. As Benner puts it, "Clinical judgment cannot be separated from ethical reasoning because each clinical judgment judges what good is at stake and what to do in each particular situation."[22]

In 2000 Benner set out what she considered to be nursing's seven moral skills:

1. relational skills in meeting the other in his or her particularity drawing on life-manifestations of trust, mercy and openness of speech;
2. perceptiveness, e.g., recognizing when a moral principle such as justice is at stake;
3. skilled know-how that allows for ethical comportment and action in particular encounters in a timely manner;
4. moral deliberation and communication skills that allow for justifications of and experiential learning about actions and decisions (Dreyfus et al. 1994);
5. an understanding of the goals or ends of good nursing practice (Rubin 1996, 191);
6. participation in a practice community that allows for character development to actualize and extend good nursing practice; and
7. the capacity to love ourselves and our neighbours, and the capacity to be loved.[23]

It is important to examine in detail the ideas and values in the above statement. The supposedly inextricable bond between clinical and ethical reasoning is a leap in logic for many. It is far from a commonplace that knowledge, excellence, even competence in any practice, need be accompanied by good, let alone exemplary, interpersonal or human skills. In fact, for most working nurses there is an often observed disconnect in such attributes in highly skilled colleagues. So how can it be argued that excellent clinical judgment is predicated on moral or ethical excellence? And, perhaps more important than the philosophical exegesis, what are the professional concerns that need to be raised over such an approach to understanding nursing expertise?

I will examine three main elements to the notion of the good in nursing as explicated by Benner: nursing as a moral practice; the recognition of the good by the good nurse; and the idea of the good as a defense against scientific and rationalist forces (medical and institutional) in health care. There are a number of significant philosophical threads that are manifest in this set of ethical imperatives. It is clearly a paradigm heavily indebted to phenomenological ideas of prereflective truths and embodied capacities, that is, the idea that there is inherent meaning and value, or truth, underlying every human situation that is independent of our knowledge of it. Free from logical analysis or any form of abstract understanding (prereflective), there is an order to the universe (God's hand) that gives purpose, meaning, and value to existence. Such a view identifies rational thought as an obstacle to understanding; rather, it is through embodied presence that "knowing," as opposed to knowledge, is possible. Other threads include the humanist reworking of the Christian concept of agape (the notable "love and be loved") and the rationalist concession to organizational skills ("a timely manner"). However, the critical thread to our discussion is the neo-Aristotelian tradition manifest in the goals of moral practice and the idea of a practice community.

Nursing as Moral Practice

In 1996 in *Expertise in Nursing Practice* Benner wrote, "We have argued that nursing practice is a form of engaged moral reasoning and that expert nurses enter care of particular patients with a fundamental sense of what is good and right."[24]

For Benner and other neo-Aristotelians, it is nursing work itself that situates it as a fundamental moral practice. She argues that it is not the individual nurse's disposition toward what is good and right that is at issue. Nor is it a matter of individual ethics. What situates nursing as a fundamentally moral practice for the neo-Aristotelians is the idea that its ethos emerges from the socially constructed and embedded ethos of the discipline, as it emerges from the ethos of practice itself. What they mean by this is that within the neo-Aristotelian God-given order of the universe, each practice has embedded within it a notion of the good—an ethical truth. This truth is independent of exterior rational formulations such as codes of ethics, rules, or principles, or at times even what the patient wants. As MacIntyre argued in the 1980s, there is an underlying "good" in nursing, medicine, teaching, architecture, and other "practices." According to MacIntyre, an activity can only be considered a practice if virtues historically flourish:

> To enter into a practice is to enter into a relationship not only with its contemporary practitioners, but also with those who have preceded us in the practice, particularly those whose achievements extended the reach of the practice to its present point. It is thus the achievement, and a fortiori the authority, of a tradition which I then confront and from which I have to learn. And for this learning and the relationship to the past which it embodies the virtues of justice, courage and truthfulness are prerequisite in precisely the

same way and for precisely the same reasons as they are in sustaining present relationships within practices.[25]

To transpose this view to nursing, Benner argues that as a "practice" in this Aristotelian sense, nursing embodies virtues (prereflectively). Moreover, these virtues of justice, courage, and truthfulness are a stable historical prerequisite for sustaining relationships within the practice. For Benner it is this situated ethic that in conjunction with the norms and mores of the nurse's unit or service, provides the "background" for the nurse's practice, and establishes it as a moral endeavor that in and of itself tends toward "the good," like a plant inclines toward the sun.

As Benner states it:

> We argue that even in clinical situations, where the ends are not in question, there is an underlying moral dimension: the fundamental disposition of the nurse towards what is good and right and action towards what the nurse recognizes or believes to be the best in a particular situation.[26]

As a set of individual precepts there is little with which to take issue here. To conceptualize nursing as a fundamentally moral act is hardly radical; it is entirely consistent with the occupation's religious origins and nineteenth-century professionalization by pious women such as Florence Nightingale. However, it may come as a surprise to some to find it embedded so squarely in contemporary conceptualizations of expertise—all the way from licensing to career pathways. And while this view may be consonant with the worldview and religious beliefs of a good many Western nurses, one must ask whether this is an appropriate stance for the profession as a whole.

The idea of the good embedded in practice is, in fact, based on an arcane but influential theological and philosophical perspective, Scholasticism, the medieval school of thought based on the work of St. Thomas Aquinas. Picking up the Aristotelian thread, Benner and her colleagues develop their argument in relation to ethical reasoning. According to Benner and her colleagues, "Authentic caring in this sense is common to Pauline agape and Aristotelian phronesis."[27] This Scholastic Aristotelian perspective (the fusion of Aristotelianism and the work of Thomas Aquinas) forges an inextricable link between ethical attributes (agape) and practice-based expertise (phronesis).

What Is Best Is Not Evident Except to the Good Nurse

The consequences of this rethinking of ethics, expertise, and skill is that it sets up nursing practice as an essentially ethical form of conduct. By doing so, clinical skill and expertise are reconstituted as an expression of exemplary ethical understanding.

For Benner, the moral agency of the nurse is fully socially embedded with better recognition of what those present in the situation can bring to it. An increased ability to read the situation allows the nurse to step in and step back as the situation demands.[28]

Critically, this ethical understanding for Benner arises unmediated from the practice domain itself. Importantly, this ethical activity is independent of any principle-based formulations. It is not based on abstractions, nor can generalizations be made across situations:

> Nursing is also—and this constitutes its total uniqueness—a domain which shows forth clearly that in some human areas there is no place at all for abstract, objective, universal theory, nor for analytic rationality. Besides being the perfect model of a craft (techne), the caring practices of nursing provide a paradigm case of skills that have no theoretical component at all.[29]

Here we have a formulation of nursing as an essentially ethical activity based on a situated skill set that is free from theoretical, intellectual, or structural determinants. It is difficult to recognize nursing practice in such a formulation. For Benner and her colleagues the correct path to the good is not only free from determined formulations or ethical codes, it may only be accessible to the expert. As Aristotle said, "What is best is not evident except to the good man" (5.1.12.259).[30] This vital element of ethical expertise, that the hidden meaning may be unclear to all except the "good" nurse, heralds a major departure from the usual mode of ethical knowledge and conduct in nursing and the professions. Even though this expert nurse may take a course of action counter to colleagues, the patient, or the patient's family, the expert's superior grasp of the context makes her the only one who understands the correct way toward the good.

In *Expertise in Nursing Practice* Benner further says, "For the expert nurse, new possibilities of moral agency are created by clinical grasp, embodied know-how, and the ability to see likely future eventualities in clinical situations."[31] This ability to see the likely future is a common theme in the expert narratives developed through Benner's research. The focus is often on the nurse's ability to recognize that something is brewing with the patient and her ability to anticipate and thus avert catastrophe. As Benner puts it, "Typically, if the nurse mentions skilled performance, it is linked with anticipating likely future events."[32]

The picture here is of expert nurses who, because of their practice knowledge, the embedded values of the discipline, and their practice context, quite simply know "the good" as it pertains to the patient, and thus act a fortiori in an ethically sound way. True experts know this in an intuitive way. It is neither based on articulated principles nor is it necessarily evident to others. In fact, it may be contrary to objective determinations, such as scientific data or ethical principles. Like a member of the Calvinist elect, the expert nurse simply knows. As opposed to the "experienced" nurse, the "expert" has confidence in her intuition to go against reason and the ability to trust her instincts as opposed to data. According to Benner, to lack this faith in intuition is to fall victim to rationalist science and to close oneself off to the practice wisdom accessible only through an embodied connection with the patient.

One of the key elements in this ethical knowledge for Benner lies in the expert nurse's recognition of the possibilities for harm in overzealous treatment and institutional rigidities, as Benner puts it, in "limiting the encroachment of technology."[33] For neo-Aristotelians, ethical expertise makes manifest this humanist sensibility to protect the patient. Although few would disagree that the protection of the patient from futile treatments or inappropriately aggressive management is an important element of nursing work, for neo-Aristotelians this particular element of ethical comportment emanates from the view that there is an irreducible gulf between the human sciences (such as nursing) and medical science.

Like Charles Taylor, Benner believes in a dualistic and antagonistic relationship between the human and the natural sciences. Nursing, as a moral practice, is thought to buffer the patient from the effects of naked instrumental reason. Benner's project, as she puts it, is to aid the "recovery" of an understanding of the nature of clinical and ethical comportment and reasoning lodged in a practice.[34] This goal is given further impetus in the juxtaposition that Benner poses, again from Taylor and MacIntyre, between the legitimacy of scientific reasoning versus the "craft, judgement, relationships and moral virtues" of clinicians.

The philosophical and theological threads that link ethical expertise with a stand against science and instrumental reason are important to this discussion. The moral and ethical superiority of nursing as a practice serves important ends for neo-Aristotelians. As adherents to the view that the human and natural sciences are essentially antagonistic, they juxtapose the legitimacy of scientific reasoning with the "craft, judgement, relationships and moral virtues" of clinicians. Benner defines moral agency for the expert nurse as centered on three features: (1) developing the skill of involvement; (2) managing technology and preventing technological intrusions; and (3) working with and through others.[35]

Rather than being based on clinical criteria, protocols, or other objective measures, these elements depend on the expert nurse's ability to resist the rational and accede to the truth underlying every situation. According to Benner, the way the expert can "break through" to the good and the right in every situation is by focusing on his or her emotions. In Benner's view, the emotional response "contains within it a vision of habits of skills, thought and relationship. Emotions are more than noise that trouble our cognitive processing; they create the possibility of rational action. Emotional responses can act as a moral compass in responding to the other person."[36] This insight is also indebted to Taylor, who argues that "the inner voice of my true sentiments defines what is the good."[37] Or, in Benner's words, "Taylor's view of the emotions as socially constituted and meaningful opens up the possibility of attuned, skillful care guided by an emotion-based understanding of the situation."[38]

Benner's expert nurses expressed in their narratives this moral imperative to buffer the patient from the effects of medical zeal. She concluded: "We found that some expert nurses shared an ethos of following the body's lead and limiting the use of technology in order to restore the patient."[39] Such narratives include examples of ensuring pain management before procedures, preparing the family and the patient for the withdrawal of treatment, and nurses' ability to change priorities as patient death approaches (focusing on family instead of pathology reports).[40] In fact, these are fairly typical clinical activities for nurses. One wonders at the value of a recategorization of these acts as examples of ethical, rather than clinical, expertise.

Moreover, there are further troubling concerns in the expansion of expertise to include ethical competence and expertise. These concerns arise from the use of narratives to also define inexpert practice—clinical and ethical—as one without an appropriate narrative. This line of reasoning by Benner and colleagues has led to the development of a novel category of practitioner. Nurses who cannot recount a particular kind of narrative are dubbed "experienced but not expert."

Experienced But Not Expert: An Ethical Failure?

As part of a study by Benner and colleagues in intensive care nursing published in 1996, Jane Rubin examined a group of nurses whose unit managers deemed them to be expert, but whom the research team considered to be "experienced" not "expert."[41] According to Benner and colleagues, the critical distinction that emerged was in the domain of moral expertise. Rubin described the defining characteristics of experienced but not expert nurses as being prone to not taking responsibility and to expressing the feeling that they were not very important.[42]

On the one hand, these nurses cannot experience themselves as doing what is good in critical clinical situations; on the other hand, they clearly have moral qualms about their actions that they cannot effectively articulate to themselves or others. As a result, they consistently attribute the responsibility for their decisions to other people.[43]

Benner supports this analysis, arguing the expert nurse's skills are demonstrated through her emotional attunement to and her suspicion of the objective, rational domain.[44] The nurse is constituted as expert through a process where she develops a repertoire of skills for engaging in practice at a level that privileges faith over reason and where she follows her well-calibrated moral compass through finely tuned emotional responses. This is not simply an opportunity for the nurse to extend her clinical range through emotional engagement, it is a prerequisite for expert practice. For Benner, "emotional attunement is central to expert clinical and ethical comportment."[45] Without an emotional compass the nurse is not expert—she will remain merely experienced. Benner makes her point by quoting Callahan, "A person who wrestles with moral questions is usually emotionally committed to doing good and avoiding evil. A good case can be made that what is specifically moral about moral thinking, what gives it its imperative 'oughtness' is personal emotional investment."[46]

In Dreyfus's view a "full" expert nurse is committed to a high level of clinical autonomy and obliged to enact this role as an independent ethical actor. The clear danger here is that we can slip into thinking of the expert nurse as a committed and participating autonomous actor, ethically and professionally. No room is provided in this construct for a nurse whose role allows for little autonomy or for one who is reluctant to fulfill such a heavy obligation to participate in ethical life. In fact the Benner position gives few concessions to the timid. As Rubin puts it, "If this nurse had acted in the way this interviewer wishes she had, she would have acted with authority. She would have felt authorized by the standards of practice to do what was best for her patient."[47] Yet at the same time Rubin notes that these nonexpert nurses "seem to find responsibility frightening."[48]

This is a value-laden critique of nurses who may be functioning at less than optimal levels. The form of practice for these nonexpert nurses is described as "one in which clinical knowledge and ethical judgement play no meaningful role in the experience of the practitioners." Further, "One of the most common themes in the interviews with these nurses is their feeling that they are not very important," and "the nurse's feeling that she made no difference in this situation, in other words, is directly related to her lack of knowledge of clinical qualitative distinctions and practices that support them."[49]

Thus it is that those nurses who stumble forward, expressing confusion, misgivings, and even unhappiness with the ways in which they, their colleagues, or the system, have failed their patients, are paradoxically dismissed as inexpert. The nurse who is deemed merely competent or experienced is not only viewed in derisory professional terms, she now appears to be morally questionable. But is this the only conclusion that can be drawn from the fact that "experienced" nurses failed to articulate their role as a particular form of ethical persona? An alternate explanation might be that those whom the authors considered to be the merely "experienced" nurses were unable to produce not expert practice but the required expert narrative. Recall that the function of Benner's clinical narratives is not a mere relating of events. Contemporary understandings of expertise rely on the production of desirable narratives that represent nursing knowledge and skill in particular ways. The narrator is engaged in selecting a particular ordering of events to construct meaning akin to the desired "point of view."[50] This blurring of clinical skill and narrative ability has produced a remarkable situation for nursing. As Mary Ellen Purkis and I have argued in relation to the regulation of nurses in Canada and the licensing requirement that nurses keep a reflective journal as evidence of competency, nurses who can talk the talk—either by writing the requisite clinical exemplar or by talking about their work in very specific ways—are viewed as providing evidence of expertise.[51] The distinction between saying and doing appears to have been lost!

This elision of saying and doing is particularly relevant in Benner and colleagues' discussion of expertise and the ethical dimension of care.[52] For ethical expertise, just as in the clinical exemplars published in the many Benner texts, the key to recognition of expert status is the construction of a narrative. As Benner defines it, the novice nurse's focus is directed at the immediate. She lacks the capacity to read the landscape like her expert colleague. For Benner the practical and ethical dimensions of this concrete, situated nursing skill are fused, and as a consequence the researcher's interpretation of the nurse's ethical capacities is colored. Because these ethical and clinical dimensions are, in this interpretative system, fundamental to a nurse's progress along the novice-to-expert continuum, the "novice" nurse may be viewed as deficient in the realms of both morality and practice.

Implications

Let us stop here to think through the implications of such a view of expertise and ethical capacity. If it is correct that embedded ethical capacity is derived from an advanced situated understanding, is not the reverse also true? Does this mean that a novice nurse is also a novice in terms of her ethical capacities? As Benner says, "But if being good means being able to learn from experience and use what one has learned so as to respond more appropriately to the demands of others in a concrete situation, the highest form of ethical comportment consists of being able to stay involved and to refines one's intuitions.[53] Without the "expert's intuitions" nurses simply have to rely on judgment or principles, a lower level of ethical capacity for Benner. The expert nurse is seen as so skilled in intuitively determining the correct ethical path that if she is in a situation in which she cannot rely on experiential precedent, she cannot be assisted by principles or guidelines but must turn to what Benner terms "detached reflection,"[54] where the nurse relies on intuitive ability, which we recall is free from principles, knowledge, or institutional data.

In Benner's view, "The practitioner must develop the moral art of attentiveness, and willingness to be with patients who are suffering." The way the expert nurse—as opposed to the experienced nurse—does this is by maintaining her confidence in her intuition to challenge reason. She relies on the infallible ability to trust her instincts as opposed to data. To lack this faith is to fall victim to rationalist science and to close oneself off to the practice wisdom accessible only through an embodied connection with the patient. It seems that fallible nurses are not expert. "The good" in this case involves, as Benner puts it, "limiting the encroachment of technology."[55] Ethical expertise, then, is what MacIntyre described as a defense against the "corrupting power of institutions." By focusing on the body and soul of the person, MacIntyre believes "humanity" prevents the objectification inherent in institutional rationality.[56]

An important difficulty with this moral high ground of ethical expertise is that it privileges one ethical style over all others. To equate nursing expert practice, in both an ethical and a clinical sense, with one form of ethical comportment renders other nurses (almost all of them) devoid of ethical capacity or expert status. Such a view fails to recognize the wide repertoire of ethical capacities that most nurses use in their daily work with vulnerable and often difficult patients (let alone with colleagues!). The professional shaping of nurses of even modest competence includes a vast array of skills that do not necessarily relate to the emotivist-humanist capacities Benner so heavily emphasizes in her care ethic.

For instance, the ability to handle difficult patients, to be kind to people one does not like, to sensitively deal with body breakdown, to joke and pass the time with patients and colleagues, and to moderate the scientific or institutional rationalities to fit the mood and the morning are scarcely out-of-reach capabilities for most nurses. Perhaps too the capacity *not* to bring the day home with you is more important than the capacity for "care ethics," with its emphasis on intense involvement. It is, in fact, highly unlikely that the "seven moral sources" of Benner's embodied life-world intersect with the everyday modes of ethical conduct adhered to by most nurses.

Moreover, this ethically expert nurse will face an increasingly difficult time in today's health care world, characterized as it is by cost-cutting and work overload. Benner and her colleagues do acknowledge the reorganization, redesign, and reengineering of health care that has taken place during the twelve years between the publication of *Novice to Expert* and *Expertise in Nursing Practice*. They flag the critical issues of nonnursing personnel, skill mix, the creation of designated acute care hospitals, and the radically new role of the manager.[57] They also acknowledge the impact of too few skilled nurses working with extremely ill patients in today's pressured health care system. Nonetheless, the concept of expertise (clinical and ethical) reaffirms the primacy of individual solutions, as opposed to systemwide responses. In Benner's work, the identification of moral and ethical behavior seems to exist in the realm of perfection, as opposed to the highly imperfect world of practice. It is the exemplary, the transcendent, and the remarkable to which her discourse is devoted. Of course the search for excellence is part of any profession's obligation to its discipline. That said, the intertwining of ethical and clinical expertise shifts this issue dramatically. If only a few remarkable nurses qualify as expert—that is, as highly skilled intuitive autonomous actors prepared to take responsibility for their actions—what does this make the rest of the profession? Are they unethical? It is hard to avoid the conclusion that, in this discourse, most nurses miss the mark.

This is where the particular theoretical and methodological position of Benner risks creating serious problems for nursing. How does it accommodate the nurse who is overwhelmed? And in truth, how many hardworking nurses, tired from shift work, mandatory overtime, juggling family responsibilities and job insecurities, are not struggling to deliver even the minimum standard of care in health systems that are cutting costs all around them? The real nurse's inability to generate an expert narrative may be more a consequence of demoralization, or class, or education than any reflection of her competence, commitment, or ethical expertise. Is all we have to offer these nurses, as Benner suggests, "consciousness raising groups . . . to address the sources of disengagement and disenchantment?"[58]

Moreover, nursing is a mass secular occupation and not all nurses worldwide believe in an intrinsic god-given truth that underlies the social and material fabric of our existence. Yet it is only from such a premise that the notion of ethical expertise makes sense. In fact, it is only through Aristotle's (and later Aquinas's) god-given order to the universe that the intuitive power of the expert exists at all. Despite the particularity of its intellectual and theological genesis, the idea of the expert nursing clinician and the five-stage model has attached itself to nursing's self-view with such power that it will doubtless be around for many years to come. Although there may be those with misgivings as to the helpfulness of this model of skill acquisition, expertise, and professional pathways,[59] the response of nurses, from students to leaders, is testimony to the resonance of the idea.

The notion of ethical expertise, however, adds a troubling dimension to this idea of clinical expertise. One must question how meaningful, let alone helpful, it is to conceptualize nursing as fundamentally moral work. Where is the purpose in reclassifying activities such as pain management, the shift to palliative care at the end of life, and family care as moral as opposed to clinical skills? When the capacity of the system to provide nurses to deliver care is seriously under threat, how helpful is it to cast nursing as essentially "good" work and to assign the better or more expert nurse to the higher moral ground? Surely, this formulation is something of a diversion in the hardheaded world of the first decade of the twenty-first century, when nursing's legitimacy rests with its ability to demonstrate its effectiveness and its critical relationship to patient outcomes.

Some might argue that this emphasis on outcomes devalues caring and that the variety of nursing activities might be difficult to quantify. However, the recent shift in discourse to a focus on patient outcomes does not mean that caring need be abandoned as a nursing imperative. How can patients do well in our pressured systems without competent, experienced, and compassionate nurses? Thanks to the last decade of research, we not only know, but can show, that they cannot.[60] But we do need to question whether their recovery, not to mention their survival, depends on the "goodness" of expert nurses more than on their competence.

Although the pursuit of excellence is the mandate of every profession, the problem with this particular idea of ethical expertise is that it places an unfair ethical load on everyday nurses. This adds to the already burdensome sense of failure that many nurses struggle against. Does the failure to achieve mastery against such odds and to voice an expert narrative render nurses inexpert and call into question their ethical integrity? Susan James's observations on the capacity to engage as an active citizen are apposite here. She argues in relation to voice, gender, and civic participation:

> Once we look more carefully, however, it is evident that the condition of speaking in one's own voice embodies a number of complexities. If I am to

speak in my own voice, I must at least see myself as having an individual voice. But this capacity rests on two further requirements. In the first place, I must see myself as separate from others, for it is otherwise difficult to see how I can grasp the idea of a voice being mine. In the second place, I must see myself as possessing a voice that is mine. For there are many ways of perceiving myself as a separate individual, yet lacking the ability to speak for myself.[61]

Benner and colleagues interpret silence and confusion, characteristics that could well be the result of professional or institutional politics in which the nurse finds it extremely difficult to find his or her voice and to perform as an autonomous moral actor, with individual rather than system-driven deficiencies. Dreyfus is clear that nurses such as those observed by Rubin during the Benner expertise-in-nursing study, nurses who failed to articulate their practice according to the narrative standard but instead expressed confusion and powerlessness in their practice, did not meet the mark in ethical attributes. He argues that "everyday intuitive ethical expertise, according to Aristotle, was formed by the sort of daily practice that produces good character."[62] But can the failure of nurses to achieve expert status in the terms of Benner and her colleagues really be reduced to a problem of character?

Sociologist Daniel Chambliss found in his study of U.S. hospitals, the ethical dilemmas that confronted and silenced nurses were scarce resources, professional rivalries, and institutional policies.[63] Chambliss was also highly skeptical about the possibility for autonomous practice by nurses. He found that the scope of practice of most nurses in his study was contained by medical directives and institutional protocols. Moreover, Chambliss observed that nurses behaved, both passively and actively, as a group and not as individual ethical actors.

Taking a very different approach in his analysis of nursing and its ethical dilemmas Chambliss observed the following:

1. nurses are not the lowest people in the hospital hierarchy but they are clearly subordinates: often ignored, shown little respect, and generally undervalued. They carry out vital work and are typically not recognized or rewarded for that. Much of their work is of low visibility and of little dramatic potential. In this their situation is typical of that of many women.

2. this is not to say nurses are morally better than doctors or anyone else. They are fundamentally employees in a helping profession. Their self-description as "patient advocates" is as much ideology as objective description.[64]

The home truths that Chambliss is pointing out contrast sharply with the ethical expertise perspective, where the individual expert nurse is apparently able to achieve her ends despite the structural limitations that confine her practice. Reducing the so-called ethical incapacity of "experienced but not expert nurses" to an individual failure silences a critical discussion of the impotence many nurses experience. Might their failure to influence patient care be as indicative of system failures as it is of their own moral insufficiency?

Chambliss's observations raise the question as to why the particular view of Benner and her colleagues on expertise has been so compelling for nurses, from bedside nurses to professors to regulators. I suggest this is due to two reasons. Primarily it is because Benner's notion of expertise wrote the idea of nursing knowledge and skill into being. It was and remains the big breakthrough for nursing scholarship and practice. With the idea of situated expertise Benner provided an exciting new path for nurses. It was a path to make visible, create a language, and begin the complex process of studying and, importantly, rewarding clinical expertise, free of the tangled and obscure nursing theory attempts of the preceding decades. For its time it was a liberating ideology. It recognized and then promoted nursing skill through the academy, through health services, and through the profession.

And yet from the beginning there were troubling elements. Embedded in the radical message of the 1970s, a time that now seems part of the golden age before managerialism and cost-cutting, was a highly romantic idea of nursing as an expression of Gilligan's "women's ways of knowing."[65] What Suzanne Gordon and I argue elsewhere in this book is that what may have been a trump card at one time, such as the construction of nursing as a feminine moral domain in the nineteenth century—a strategy that enabled women to leave the patriarchal home and move into the workplace and play a significant role in society—becomes a liability in another context.[66] Although it makes nurses feel special, the moral high ground may inadvertently serve to lower the value of nursing in contemporary society, where success is increasingly measured in terms of prestige and tax bracket. Nurses may do well in most polls that measure trust, but nursing ranks poorly as a desirable career for intelligent and motivated men and women.[67] The idea that a good nurse is ipso facto a good person, and that good practice is an essentially moral act, once again obscures what nurses know and do. This overarching discourse on nurses as moral agents simply reasserts what Gordon and I have termed the "virtue script."

The idea of the expert nurse as one who embodies ethical expertise may similarly take nurses and nursing in a direction that provides little ammunition for the hard battles nurses need to fight to maintain standards of patient care. How many nurses feel the power and the certainty of Benner's experts today? If self-doubt and the inability to articulate the moral dimension of failing standards renders us experienced but not expert, we must surely be in the good company of a great many nurses and physicians working today.

What are the alternatives for conceptualizing a more realistic view of what nurses do and know? Can we not abandon the idea of "the good" as a truth that underpins all human (and cosmic) activity? And where, as Weber would have put it, is the "natural home" of nursing ethics if it is neither in the caring domain of agape, phronesis, and intuition nor in the uncaring rationalist world of biomedical models?

Perhaps the answer to that question lies in our reference point. If our starting point in discussing both ethics and expertise is, for once, not situated in the realm of principles or exemplary narratives, but in everyday collective practice, we may be able to bring into focus the more modest, but no less powerful, ethical capacities through which nurses habitually enact their practice. Whether they are expert in an ideal or transcendent sense is entirely the wrong question. Rather we need to examine nurses' abilities to function within an increasingly dysfunctional system.

As a profession we need to grapple with acknowledging the clinical knowledge and skill of nurses and to be comfortable in the scientific and medico-technical realm in which so much excellent nursing is practiced. In the end it is what nurses do, not what nurses say about what they do, that makes the difference in patient care. Talking the talk is no substitute for walking the walk, and measures of expertise certainly need a sounder basis than elicited practice narratives. The idea of ethical expertise brings home the perils of confusing doing and saying, and it highlights the risks to nursing if we persist in subjugating clinical knowledge and skill to the idea of nursing as a moral practice. Perhaps we should listen more closely to the so-called experienced but not expert narratives. They tell us a story we do not wish to hear. It is not a story of ethical triumph but of the harsh daily reality of working nurses from Sydney to San Francisco, from long-term care to coronary care. It is the story of nurses feeling overwhelmed, of not knowing what to do let alone how to do it better, as the system stretches, and sometimes snaps, around them. It is the story of nurses dealing with the situation the best ways they can, some better than others, some days better than others. It is a story that needs to be acknowledged.

6

From Sickness to Health

Tom Keighley

This chapter considers the forty-year journey that nursing began at the World Health Assembly in 1978 with the Declaration of Alma-Ata and its universally adopted target "Healthcare for All—2000."[1] It is an attempt to throw some light on why nurses, at least in their public pronouncements, appear to have moved away from the care of sick people and now focus so intently on purveying information about how to stay well. For many nurses and their organizations this change in focus from sickness to health underpins their strategies for the promotion of their profession. During this period, nursing has moved from being the handmaiden of the doctor to something resembling a self-standing profession, a considerable achievement. However, in embracing the concept of health and diminishing the significance of the care of the sick, nursing has run the risk of leaving the sick patient behind.

In launching a major critique of the illness and medicalized focus of health care the Declaration of Alma-Alta moved the emphasis away from acute illness to something as yet undetermined—health. In doing so, it redefined the role of nurses involved in health care. Rather than emphasizing the work of the care of the sick that most nurses were, and are, engaged in, the declaration and nurses' embrace of its fundamental philosophy has helped conceal the importance of sickness and the importance of nurses' work managing illness. In this essay I ask whether nursing's choices and organizational positioning have left the sick dangerously exposed. To answer this question, I consider when this change occurred, what motivated it, its impact on nursing, and its implications.

Repositioning Nursing

If one listens to nurses talk about their work or examines the mission statements of nursing organizations, it is clear that nursing has, at least rhetorically, increasingly removed itself from the care of the sick.

For decades, nurses have engaged in an ongoing exercise in how to define and position their work to gain social legitimacy and value. One of the most important actors in this effort has been the International Council of Nurses (ICN), which was founded in 1899. The ICN set out to give nurses global networks for communication and to promote the status of the nurse. It now represents nurses in over 120 countries and undertakes work on nursing practice, nursing regulation, and the social and economic welfare of nurses. As well as drawing the profession together and supporting the advancement of nurses and nursing practice, it works to influence health policy all over the world.

To gain the kind of recognition that has long been denied the nursing profession, in the 1950s the ICN engaged in a round of debates with national nurses' associations about a definition of nursing. It retained consultant Virginia Henderson to lead this work. Henderson came to prominence in the United States because of her interest in establishing a research base for nursing practice. She formulated her definition of nursing as part of the revision of Bertha Harmer's *Textbook of the Principles and Practice of Nursing*. Her work was driven by a desire to distinguish between the work of doctors and nurses, as well as to distinguish the role of informal caregivers from the professionalism of the registered nurse. The definition the ICN adopted was similar to Henderson's 1955 definition of nursing:

> Nursing is primarily helping people (sick or well) in the performance of those activities contributing to health, or its recovery (or to a peaceful death) that they would perform unaided if they had the necessary strength, will, or knowledge. It is likewise the function of nurses to help people gain independence as rapidly as possible.[2]

Although Henderson's definition of nursing contains a host of cultural assumptions that largely went unchallenged, in 1960 the ICN settled on this definition:

> Nursing is primarily assisting individuals (sick or well) in the performance of those activities contributing to health, or its recovery (or to a peaceful death) that they would perform unaided if they had the necessary strength, will, or knowledge. Nursing is a process through which care is provided to individuals, families, or groups.[3]

The major difference between the definitions is that nursing is, in the ICN definition, a service for families and groups as well as individuals. Placed in a different political and social context, this expands the role of the nurse into social engagement beyond the existing role of carer for the sick. This definition has been revised several times. The latest ICN definition (2002) reads:

> Nursing encompasses autonomous and collaborative care of individuals of all ages, families, groups and communities, sick or well and in all settings. Nursing includes the promotion of health, prevention of illness, and the care of the ill, disabled and dying people. Advocacy, promotion of a safe environment, research, participation in shaping health policy and in patient health systems management, and education are also key nursing roles.[4]

Though some forty years separate these two definitions, their common ancestry is obvious both in the language used and sentiments expressed. Although Henderson retained the original ethos of nursing by referring to "sick or well" in that order, the ICN definition equates the two states. Giving equal valance to health and illness sets the stage for significant subsequent changes in nursing's self-definition. Indeed, the current ICN definition reflects more fully the desire of nurses to be seen as a separate profession whose functions include health promotion, disease avoidance, advocacy, research, policy formulation, and education. The leadership position of the ICN is reflected in the mission statements of nurses' organizations around the world. Statements from four influential nurses' organizations demonstrate this.

The Australian Nursing Council's *Code of Professional Conduct for Nurses in Australia* is the statement of a regulatory body that holds legal powers to impose its decisions on registered nurses in Australia. It states that the nurse must:

1. Practise in a safe and competent manner
2. Practise in accordance with the agreed standards of the profession
3. Nor bring discredit upon the reputation of the nursing profession
4. Respect the dignity, culture, values and other beliefs of an individual and any significant other person
5. Support the health, well-being and informed decision-making of an individual
6. Promote and preserve the trust that is inherent in the privileged relationship between a nurse and an individual, and respect both the person and property of that individual
7. Treat personal information obtained in a professional capacity as confidential

8. Refrain from engaging in exploitation, misinformation and misrepresentation in regard to health care products and nursing services.[5]

Each of these statements is then elaborated on, but, remarkably, at no point are the key words of patient, illness, or sickness used. The patient has become the individual, sometimes receiving care and sometimes not. The code reflects the profession's modern concern to be open to all aspects of social activity that might conceivably be claimed as part of a nurse's work. From this code it is impossible to determine where the boundaries of professional nursing practice begin and end.

The Canadian Nurses Association (CNA) takes this dynamic one step further by using a set of values as its Code of Ethics:

CNA believes the following eight values are central to nursing practice.

1. Safe, Competent, and Ethical Care. Nurses value the ability to provide safe, competent and ethical care that allows them to fulfill their ethical and professional obligations to the people they serve.

2. Health and Well-Being. Nurses value health promotion and well-being and assisting persons to achieve their optimum level of health in situations of normal health, illness, injury, disability or at the end of life.

3. Choice. Nurses respect and promote the autonomy of persons and help them to express their health needs and values and also to obtain desired information and services so that they can make informed decisions.

4. Dignity. Nurses recognize and respect the inherent worth of each person and advocate for respectful treatment of all persons.

5. Confidentiality. Nurses safeguard information learned in the context of a professional relationship, and ensure it is shared outside the health care team only with the person's informed consent, or as may be legally required, or where the failure to disclose would cause significant harm.

6. Justice. Nurses uphold principles of equity and fairness to assist persons in receiving a share of health services and resources proportionate to their needs and in promoting social justice.

7. Accountability. Nurses are answerable for their practice, and they act in a manner consistent with their professional responsibilities and standards of practice.

8. Quality Practice Environments. Nurses value and advocate for practice environments that have the organizational resources necessary to ensure safety, support and respect for all persons in the work setting.[6]

In this catalog of activities and obligations, the organization never mentions patients. In a list of other issues, there is one reference to illness and one to disability. Rather than taking guidance from the realities of caring for sick people, it draws its legitimacy from a wide range of sources external to nursing and clearly places a priority on health work with informed consumers and rational choice makers.

The world's largest national nurses' association, the Royal College of Nursing (RCN) in the United Kingdom, has also spent years producing a statement defining nursing. Although the work remains unfinished, the draft documents are of great importance, because the Royal College of Nursing is one of the few nurses' organizations that emphasizes what nurses do, that is, nursing. Its current draft defines nursing as

> the use of clinical judgement in the provision of care to enable people to improve, maintain, or recover health, to cope with health problems, and to achieve the best possible quality of life, whatever their disease or disability, until death.[7]

Before identifying six defining characteristics, the opening statement carries a rare reference to disease, but there is no reference to patients. Its attempts to identify the uniqueness of nursing appear under the headings of purpose, intervention, domain, focus, value base, and commitment to partnership. The document is now over twenty pages long, and, at this writing, work on further refining has been on going for three years. That alone shows the difficulties involved. Although the document—which includes efforts to describe the unique role and contribution of nurses to health care and emphasizes the significance of education, research, and policy contributions—will impose no legal obligations on nurses, it will act as a formidable negotiating tool for the RCN in its discussion with government and employers for greater resources and enhanced status for nurses.

Finally, it is worth quoting the Vision and Mission statements of Sigma Theta Tau, the world's leading honor society for nurses. Sigma Theta Tau claims three hundred thousand members worldwide, making their mission statement juxtaposing health and knowledge of critical importance. As Sigma states it, the organization has "A Vision to Lead: To create a global community of nurses who lead in using scholarship, knowledge and technology to improve the health of the world's people." And it also has "A Mission to Serve, Support and Improve: Sigma Theta Tau International Honor Society of Nursing provides leadership and scholarship in practice, education and research to enhance the health of all people. We support the learning and professional development of our members, who strive to improve nursing care worldwide."[8] In these two statements, the explicit link between health and knowledge is central to the role of nurses involved in scholarship. This is significant because nurses who engage in scholarship are charged with fostering the next generation of nurses. Yet no mention is made of traditional concerns with sickness and illness or of patients. Although caring is mentioned in the last line of the mission statement, it contains no echo of the nature of nursing before the 1978 Declaration of Alma-Ata, which encouraged nurses to develop a knowledge base they could put into practice as a way of legitimizing nursing and giving status to nurses who care for the sick.

Whether the organization is a statutory regulatory body, a professional association, or an elite academic society, the focus is the same. The profession no longer emphasizes the suffering of the vast majority of the people nurses care for; it is concerned with health and with opportunities to promote nurses and their status. Although one can argue that there is a logical link between improving the status of nurses and improving the care of patients, none of the organizations makes that link in the documents that exist to promote the status of nurses to the public.

The significance of the focus on health seems to have been missed by many nurses and nursing organizations. Few have challenged a process that is not only connected to the profession's status and to the individual nurse's status and remuneration but, most important, to the fate of the patients nurses care for.

Sickness to Health—the Drivers for Change

Although the nursing profession's view of its own mission has been influenced by many factors, none is more important than the Declaration of Alma-Ata in its rhetorical abandonment of the care of the sick and the embrace of the pursuit of health. Developed and passed by the World Health Assembly in 1978, it challenged two unsupportable myths in health care. The first was that all health care must be, and can only be, delivered by a doctor. The second was that the only place where health care can be delivered is in a hospital. Driven by the "Two-thirds World," in contrast to the "one-third" developed world, it was both a response to economically unsupportable high-cost and high-tech medicine and to the potential of primary health care teams and community care. Widely welcomed in many countries in the world, Alma-Ata spawned a number of regional charters as countries and larger international groupings united to achieve the changes it recommended. It has also given much-needed attention to public health and the social determinates of health.

The Declaration of Alma-Ata was the culmination of 150 years in which the medical profession had brought scientific approaches to care to the fore. Considered in broad terms, before 1950 illness was perceived as episodic, with marked beginnings and ends, even if the end was death. To receive health care on a continuous basis was a new idea, arising from the successful treatment of conditions such as bacterial infections, diabetes, asthma, and schizophrenia, which responded to therapies that became widespread in the 1950s and 1960s. The nineteenth century had seen constant developments in the state of scientific and medical knowledge—particularly in surgical interventions. Although the development of anesthesia was key in this evolution, it was the recognition of the value of antibiotics, endocrine supplements, and the regular use of tranquilizers that heralded the age of scientific medicine.

This last stage of the medical revolution was characterized not only by the availability of effective therapies for certain previously unmanageable diseases but the development of the infrastructure to support them. The increasing sophistication of epidemiology, microbiology, and radiography meant that diagnosis no longer rested absolutely on the clinical observations of the doctor or nurse. Technology was available to support the decision-making process. Going hand in hand with this shift were marked improvements in the equipment available to deliver care. The importance of doing things quickly was also recognized, with specialist services to collect patients and move them into the care environment as quickly as possible. By the 1970s most of these developments were widely available in most Western countries, which began to focus on acute illness and interventions.

Although much in the Alma-Ata declaration is constructive and important, it is based on a definition of health that is both problematic and of critical importance for nursing. Section I states:

> The Conference strongly reaffirms that health, which is a state of complete physical, mental and social well-being, and not merely the absence of disease or infirmity, is a fundamental human right and that the attainment of the highest possible level of health is a most important world-wide social goal whose realization requires the action of many social and economic sectors in addition to the health sector.

For nursing and patients the key words in this statement are "merely" and "complete." Health is "is a state of complete physical, mental and social well-being," and "not merely the absence of disease or infirmity." The thrust of the simple qualifier "merely" could not be more significant. Though it went unrecognized at the time, this formulation triggered a fundamental shift in thinking about the function and position of nursing.

Sickness, disease, and infirmity, concerns that had been—and still are— central, were now a minor concern, in favor of health promotion and disease prevention. Of course, such objectives are eminently laudable. In many industrialized nations, health care systems are far too focused on acute illness and interventions rather than on chronic illness and public health. When this acute care approach is adopted by less-developed nations with few economic resources, the problematic becomes scandalous.

Because of the elevation of health over illness, all health care professionals, including nurses, were asked to refocus their mission and to construct a hierarchy of goals for their professions. To be involved in disease prevention was not "merely" doing something but was undertaking a more important function than caring for sick people. Not only did this give much-needed status to those who worked in public health, it has, over the years, removed status from those who cared for sick people. It also paves the way for stigmatizing sick people, who are no longer viewed as victims of an inevitable part of the human condition but as people who have failed to maintain their own health or prevent their own illnesses. The consequences of this move have yet to be fully realized.

The Alma-Ata declaration not only focused on freedom from disease and episodic illness and, for the patient, the diagnosable, and hopefully treatable, condition. It also considerably expanded the definition of health, moving far beyond the traditional emphasis in public health on clean water and good nutrition as fundamental to good health. Instead, clinicians and policymakers now judge whether their client's "complete" life is in harmony and whether they have attained "complete physical, mental and social well-being." This is because the declaration states that "the highest possible level of health is a most important world-wide social goal."

The declaration put the achievement of health at the top of the agendas of individuals and organizations. In so doing, it attempted to redefine something indefinable and immeasurable—the purpose of life. The goal was no longer the pursuit of happiness but of wellness or, as it began to be called, "well-being." Perhaps this is why there was no reference to the spiritual in the Alma-Ata declaration. Health, or wellness, replaced happiness or spiritual completeness in this model of what it means to be human.

Although holistic health seemed to flow from this position, the reframing of illness may actually compromise the search for holism. Rather than placing an equal emphasis on the care of the sick, as we've seen, some organizations either ignore sickness or make it of secondary importance, subordinate to health. Health care services have new goals, as do individuals, whose expectations concerning their own lives and the services available to support them have been redefined.

Because it delineates a hierarchy of significance that redefines the place of illness in the lives of individuals and in the mission of health care professionals, Alma-Ata was not simply a pivotal moment in the understanding of public health. It was also a pivotal moment for nursing.

As an all-medical or physician-only affair, nursing organizations were not invited to participate in the discussions that led to the declaration. Nonetheless, because it coincided with two significant changes in nursing, nurses' organizations were at the forefront of promoting this change. The first was the almost global implementation of care planning (also known as the nursing process), which had emerged in the United States and had been supported by World Health Organization regional offices worldwide. This was the point at which nursing practice engaged with its emerging knowledge base in determining patterns of care.

The second change occurred in the major nurses' associations. In the developed world, organizations such as the American Nurses Association, the Royal College of Nursing, the Canadian Nurses Association, and the Danish Nurses Organisation (perhaps the four most influential national associations at the time) adopted overt political positions on the health care agenda. In that context, an international declaration that supported change in responsibilities and roles became an invaluable tool. The shift in focus from hospital to community, and from illness to health, justified a redefinition of the zones of responsibility and consequence importance of nurses as health care practitioners. Nursing organizations believed that this change would not only serve the greater good of patients; they also understood that this repositioning of health care priorities could enhance the profession's status.

It is only when seen historically that the importance of the 1978 Alma-Ata declaration to nurses' subsequent embrace of some of its fundamental tenets can be recognized. We can see this in the way the declaration has been integrated into subsequent documents. The Fifty-First World Health Assembly in 1998 included on its agenda a review of the Alma-Ata declaration. The first section of that new declaration reads:

> We, the Member States of the World Health Organisation (WHO), reaffirm our commitment to the principle enunciated in its Constitution that the enjoyment of the highest attainable standard of health is one of the fundamental rights of every human being; in doing so, we affirm the dignity and worth of every person, and the equal rights, equal duties and shared responsibilities of all for health.

The right has been changed from "health" to "the highest attainable standard of health." It also emphasizes the significance of the right by describing health as "one of the *fundamental* rights." The declaration of the right to health care is, however, more complex that it seems. It does not give one the right to health care services and to care when one is sick. It gives one the right to help avoiding getting sick. When one examines how this avoidance is to be achieved, we see how problematic this is.

The 1998 statement does not deny the existence of other rights but relegates them to a second order of concern. It has to be assumed that in the presence of competition between a first order "fundamental" right and something classified as "merely the absence of disease or illness" the "merely" requirements might be ignored in certain circumstances. Not only has sickness been jettisoned in favor of health but we now have an obligation, or social expectation, to attain the highest standard of health. Further, it makes the achievement of this state a duty and responsibility for everyone.

This globalist approach makes health care the central component of life. It helps those who desire to pursue health to negotiate and demand their "rights," while removing illness and suffering even further from the agenda.

Such a Panglossian approach was bound to produce a reaction. Jill Palmer, a former health editor of one of Britain's most widely read newspapers, recently expressed some of the fundamental problems that have emerged as the public debate on rights and responsibilities is back at the top of the National Health Service agenda: "You eat, drink and smoke too much and generally enjoy the good life. You always mean to exercise but somehow you can never quite find the time. Your behaviour is foolish, but does it mean you should be denied medical care?"[9] Palmer reminds us that "there are those who cannot uphold obligations to be responsible for their health, either through poverty or lack of knowledge or cost of travel to places where cheap food or exercise opportunities are available." She warns that the British government may take the position that availability of care may determine people's compliance with advice on how to stay healthy and concludes, "You cannot be responsible for your own health when you do not know how to."

Although Palmer, like many others who believe in the wisdom of prevention and health maintenance, acknowledges that everyone would benefit from the greater adoption of health care advice guidance, she also recognizes the gap between rhetoric and reality. Although she doesn't delve into the subject, this has also a created a gap between the expectations of the public and the professionals who are supposed to serve them.

Nurses are increasingly trained to focus on health and its maintenance. The professional narrative, used to justify the work of nurses, increasingly does not mention care of the sick. As Palmer points out, though, the ordinary individual does not want to know much about that unless there is a threat to their health. Put simply, the sick want to be cared for while health care professionals want to focus on helping people not to become sick.

The focus on the pursuit of health also threatens to create another problematic fracture in both nurses' practice and self-understanding. Because of inequalities in health, the emphasis on disease avoidance and health promotion has only really been picked up by the wealthiest in first-world communities. For many of the wealthiest members of society, holistic health has become an obsession, an obsession they have the time and resources to pursue. The least well-off, on the other hand, continue to struggle to acquire even basic access to treatment. They hardly have the resources to adopt the best advice on diet or exercise. This is true of poor people in both undeveloped and highly developed countries. Perversely, therefore, the rich can become healthier because of their access to resources and information—everything from the personal trainer to organic supermarket food—while the less well-off, who have access to neither, experience a diminishing ratio of benefits. If nurses embrace the rhetoric of health, do they risk becoming inadvertent advocates of a two-tiered health care system in which health services are not available to an entire population but only an elite of wealthy individuals?

This stigmatizing of the sick has produced a backlash against the sick as the new narrative of health care transforms the right to health into a duty to stay healthy. This reproduces a problem that was first addressed by Florence Nightingale, who would have been astounded that care for the sick could be so easily dismissed. Despite her lifelong espousal of the principles of hygiene, she would have expected all available knowledge to be dedicated to the care of the sick. She constantly argued against the view that the poor were the cause of their own pauperism. Yet we once again find that the sick are held responsible for their own suffering. If illness is now considered avoidable, when people have the misfortune to be ill they are now deemed to have brought it on themselves and thus to deserve it.

These beliefs justify patterns of cost-containment and expenditure that are lower than universal care for all sick people would require. They legitimate not addressing some disease problems, such as AIDS/HIV epidemics in the poorest countries, or particular disease problems in the poorest parts of towns in developed countries, such as asthma in some children associated with poverty.

Because sickness is often seen as a failure to uphold one's duties in a rights-based paradigm, nurses need to consider some other implications of this reframing. For example, the focus on health may make it ever more difficult to get the necessary political majorities to sustain health care systems that take care of the sick as well as provide advice to those who want to stay healthy. Traditionally, sick people were able to surrender themselves to the care of others, especially when they found themselves without the resources and knowledge to cope with their condition. Today, the sick are expected to be their own negotiators or advocates. But how can they successfully do this when they often lack not just knowledge of the condition from which they suffer but also of the administrative workings of the health care system. Similarly, they often lack the kind of intellectual and economic resources available to those who are wealthier.

Because sick people are invariably too ill to take part in debates about the allocation of health care resources, they become an excluded minority. That a decision is made for them may be of little consolation to those who may not have had a part in such a debate and, when rendered dependent by illness, are in no position to negotiate or advocate for themselves.

The Impact on Nursing

How has nursing responded to this paradigm shift? It is not clear that the profession is alert to the significance of the shift. The fundamental nature of this change is, however, beginning to emerge in complaints by older nurses that newer nurses, though better educated, have much to learn in the early months of their employment about looking after people who are ill. In Britain, the RCN's 2004 congress was dominated by a report suggesting that modern nurses were too "posh" to bathe patients.

Certainly at ward level, traditional practices such as bed-bathing, serving food and drink, and bed making are now performed almost entirely by nurse assistants. A nurse's status seems to be determined by the combined factors of remoteness from routine human touch and the use of specialist skills. The more skilled a nurse, the less she or he is likely to be seen fetching a bedpan for a patient. Instead of talking about the skills involved in their hands-on care of the patient, more educated nurses will now highlight their application of negotiating or advocacy skills to negotiating, advocating for, or managing the patient's journey through the health care system. These skilled nurses use the same kind of language found in the position statements of the nursing organizations, and depict themselves as specialists in health maintenance and disease prevention. Though nursing has long argued that greater education and skill will directly benefit the patient because it will produce better bedside care, ironically the acquisition of academic excellence and advanced knowledge may not produce that benefit. Instead, in today's health care system those caregivers who have the most sustained, direct contact with the patient are less skilled workers.

Organizationally, the picture is equally interesting. The codes quoted at the beginning of this chapter demonstrate where the professional bodies and some trade unions think nursing should be placed. In this they seem to align themselves with elected officials who are intent on cutting costs. The risk is that the public will read nursing's commitment to the health agenda as part of the cost-cutting approach to health care.

If nursing has aligned itself with this move away from sickness—and funding the care of the sick–and toward a definition of health that stigmatizes the sick, this carries many risks. The pursuit of an exclusive nursing knowledge base and professional status may have blinded many nurses to the fact that professional status can't be advanced without considering what the public wants from nurses as well as the work that most nurses actually do.

The Human Components of Caring

Do most members of the public want nurses to abandon their expertise in the delivery of care to the sick in favor of the health agenda? What the public, or at least those members of the public who become patients, want is people who can take care of them when they are sick. If one takes Britain as an example, one sees this demand in the reintroduction of matrons (nursing directors of the old-school mould) into the hospital services in 2000. The decision was made neither by the profession nor by the policy advisers in the Department of Health but as a political initiative from the Prime Minister's Office following feedback from focus groups, a response to public concern about the health services. The decision reflected a traditional view that someone in the service should be responsible for those who were ill in the hospital, focusing on such concerns as hygiene, infection control, nutrition, and nursing practice.

Just as the demand for matrons showed public concern for sickness and its consequences, the response of nursing organizations shows how detached some have become from the public perception of what is important about nurses and nursing. Instead of using the matron to raise the profile of patient care, nurses in hospital management have seen the role as a way of further improving the efficiency of the service rather than its effectiveness. Rather than being in charge of hospitals most matrons are now responsible for bed-usage and early discharge regimes. Their knowledge of operational systems has been put to corporate use rather than to benefit the patients.

Another problem with this representation of nursing as focused on health is that it doesn't accurately portray what the vast majority of nurses actually do. In one way or another, most nurses are involved in the care of the sick. But all the contemporary recastings of nurses as health workers leave that out. How do nurses, and the public, feel when the bedside nurse is rendered invisible because of the new focus on health? Moreover, given the kind of caseloads nurses now carry all over the world, even if they want to do education in health maintenance and disease prevention, they have little time to do it. Is the Alma-Ata vision doomed to failure—at least for the care of the sick—because it defines the nursing profession by what it has increasingly little opportunity to do?

Alma-Ata raises another interesting question for the nursing profession. Nurses often criticize the medicalization of life, in which an increasing number of human dilemmas become medical conditions, which in turn allows doctors to invade every corner of human life. Alma-Ata's focus on health and harmony integrates nurses into a new and problematic social dynamic.

Rather than enhancing the status of nursing, one must ask whether these developments have lowered the status of nurses who deliver direct care to the sick. Why, given this shift, and the public commitment of nursing to the health rather than the illness agenda, have the pay and conditions of nurses failed to improve? Could support of the health agenda mean that nurses have lost their biggest bargaining chip—their care the sick?

Although many will welcome the notion that no group should be above criticism, the danger that has emerged is that health care professionals have no special position of regard. Nurses, even more than doctors, are likely to be attacked at work in Britain. This is now such a serious issue that week after week campaigns are being launched to try and protect health care staff from physical and verbal abuse. Could this dramatic shift from being almost untouchable to being a visible and available target of popular angst and violence result from a public belief that nurses have abandoned them, that they are "too posh to care"?

One of the undefined but quintessential notions in nursing is "tender, loving care," often abbreviated to TLC, the unconditional acceptance of an individual placed in a dependent position in the health care system, who requires something other than what the doctor has prescribed for them. Many, if not most, doctors (and other health care professionals) know that this is essential to help an individual recover from his or her illness. They also know that, while they have a part to play in this, the profession of nursing exists as the specialist resource for the delivery of this component of health care.

As a process, it consists of a number of ill-defined components, sometimes referred to as moderated love.[10] First, it acknowledges the essential humanity of an individual, no matter what they may or may not have done.

This becomes more difficult when the framing of health care condemns those who fail to adhere to the highest goals of health maintenance. The professional code of nurses requires them to respect the individual, no matter what the rest of society may feel, think, or do. Second, they are prepared to touch that person. This is no simple matter. In a society that places increasing emphasis on the integrity of one's personal space, to be a member of a profession equipped to enter, and thus potentially violate, that personal space is a crucial function. Even more so is the ability to perform the most intimate functions for someone who is ill, when they are incapable of doing it for themselves. This ability reflects a tenderness that is increasingly rare in daily life.

Third, nurses' caring work is characterized by a focus on the present moment. This does not deny the importance of achieving change in the future, but a sick person's ability to move into the future is dependent on the vital role the nurse plays in helping that person survive the present. Holding a patient's hand, in silence and in the dark of night, may be the most important factor effecting recovery. At that moment, the patient knows that in a particular way they are loved enough for someone to surrender their independence and come and share those moments of suffering.

Such caring is invariably backed up with deep and extensive technical knowledge and sophisticated plans for care delivery, but the moment of care is fundamentally human. When an individual is ill, it is their humanity that is challenged. They cannot continue to be the human being they were previously. To be in contact with people who sustain their humanity is central to the process of caring. It enables individuals to reacquire their previous humanity or adjust to another state of humanity that will enable them to continue their lives. For those in the end stage of their lives, the constant confirmation of their importance as human beings, no matter what happens, is usually the component of care that enables them and their family to adjust to the situation. It is rarely the doctor who sits holding the hand of the dying patient, or lays out their body afterward. That is the privilege of the nurse. If this process is now set within a strongly rationalistic and scientific framework, based on rights and health, the essential contradiction becomes clear.

In our modern world, it is often unpalatable to acknowledge the limitations of medical therapy. It is even more uncomfortable to acknowledge the need for a particular profession, nursing, that still retains its emphasis on serving the sick. Nursing has had a difficult time articulating the expertise involved in its work. Its failure to develop mechanisms to share the expertise involved in the humane care of the sick has not helped other health care professions and the decision makers to understand the importance of nursing. But the health rhetoric may further conceal, and thus diminish, the expertise and knowledge that is involved in this work. The health rhetoric renders it an even more hidden part of the process that has enabled the focus to move from care to cure. This is why nursing needs to consider the problems—as well as the promise—of health more systematically.

Public policy has shifted the emphasis from illness to health, and the consequences of this are just becoming visible. As the shortage of nurses becomes a global issue and not just something for the developed world to worry about, it may be possible to refocus nursing on a renewed concern about sick people. If not, we may be completing the cycle Florence Nightingale noted and fought against. The wealthy can be cared for and the poor blamed for their illness, rights or no rights! Is this what nursing wants to support?

7

The New Cartesianism

Dividing Mind and Body and
Thus Disembodying Care

Suzanne Gordon

When I began writing about nursing in the late 1980s, I embarked on a long educational journey that was to be as surprising as it was enlightening. I was not a nurse and knew very little about nursing at first. When I heard nurses discuss their work, I was both moved and attracted by their emphasis on caring, compassion, and human connection. I'd had many personal and professional encounters with the medical system and knew how impersonal it could be and how brusque doctors often appeared. The fact that the nurses' role was so often presented as a humanistic haven in a heartless medical world was thus very appealing.

When I began to observe nurses practice their profession, I quickly realized that the caring they so often described in emotional and relational terms was actually far more complex. Spending day after day with nurses, I was, of course, impressed by their emotional skills. I was, however, equally impressed by their knowledge of diseases and their treatment, and of medications and their correct administration and impact. Over the years, I have come to appreciate that much of nursing is about managing and tempering the risks patients run when they are sick, when they are treated for sickness, and when they are trying to live their lives while they are sick and undergoing medical treatment.

In my book about nurses at Boston's Beth Israel Hospital, *Life Support: Three Nurses on the Front Lines*, I described nursing as a tapestry of care, a tapestry that, to me, includes emotional, physical, intellectual, domestic, technological, and medical activities.[1] Most of us who are not nurses usually know about the caring, compassion, and kindness nurses demonstrate.

Just as I failed to appreciate the value of nursing before I began working at Beth Israel, what most people don't know is that nurses have a lot of medical knowledge as well as technical skills. The public does not know that nurses participate in the construction of medical diagnoses, often make medication recommendations, and administer and implement treatments. We know they are kind, but most of us don't know that nurses are also smart, persistent, and tough-minded.

Several anecdotes illustrate the public's limited understanding of nursing care. In *Life Support*, I wrote about an oncology nurse in a hematology-oncology clinic at what was then Beth Israel Hospital in Boston. In several chapters, I described the way this nurse administered chemotherapy to her patients. When the manuscript was finished, I sent it to a friend who is a lawyer. About a week after receiving the manuscript she called me to tell me she loved the book, that almost everything in it rang true. Of course, the nurses were wonderfully caring and attentive. "But Suzanne, you'd better go back and read what you wrote about that oncology nurse," she counseled.

"Why?" I asked.

"Because you've got it all wrong," she warned. "In your book," she continued, "the nurse is administering chemotherapy treatments and managing patients' nausea and vomiting. Nurses don't do that, that's what the doctor does."

When I was doing radio and TV appearances to publicize *Life Support*, I would often get the same response from the journalists interviewing me. It was no surprise to them that nurses were caring and compassionate. But knowledgeable and lifesaving? As one journalist commented on a national radio show, "You know what's so surprising about your book is that nurses know so much about diseases and medications." I responded that what was surprising was that she was surprised.

As I've reflected on those comments and listened to nurses talk about their work for the past fifteen years, I have to reconsider my response. Given the way nurses and nursing organizations describe nursing work and nurses' caring—often referred to as the "essence of nursing"—it would be not only surprising but astonishing if patients, family members, hospital administrators, policymakers, politicians, or journalists recognized that nurses know a lot about diseases, medications, and treatment. It would be almost miraculous if members of the public understood that nurses play a role in cure as well as care; that they treat the body, not just the mind; that they do lifesaving, not simply soul-saving work; and that they have brains, not just hearts.

One reason people know so little about nursing is that journalists and policymakers pay very little attention to the work of nurses and recycle stereotypical images about the profession. Nurses complain vociferously about their own invisibility. Unfortunately, many of their descriptions of their work detach the emotional and psychosocial from the physical, medical, and technical activities in which they, as nurses, participate.

Nurses often talk about the need to link the mind and body. They complain—and rightly so—about the reductionism in medicine and assert that, particularly when compared with physicians, they are holistic caregivers. When, however, one listens to nurses talk about their work, one is struck by a new kind of Cartesianism and reductionism that has become rampant in nursing education, nursing organizations, and that is, in turn, expressed by individual nurses. Rather than joining the body and mind, the physical and emotional, the medical and technical into that tapestry I described, nurses constantly counterpose the technical and medical with the caring, emotional, and relational. This dichotomization is one of the distinguishing characteristics of nursing discourse in the late twentieth and early twenty-first centuries.

The discussion and analysis in this chapter is based on over fifteen years of work with nurses. During this period, I have attended dozens of nursing conferences and listened to hundreds of nurses talk about their work. In workshops and classes I have conducted all over the world I have asked working nurses and nursing students, at both the undergraduate and graduate level, to relate or write short narratives describing why their work is important to patients. I have talked with nursing leaders and analyzed the messages delivered in nursing-image campaigns and in submissions that candidates prepare for clinical excellence awards. I have also interviewed nurses from a variety of countries. Here's what I've found.

Ask a nurse to describe her work or a nursing organization to describe nursing and you get a heavy emphasis on caring, holism, and the relational. While this rendition of the work of the nurse is certainly a critical part of the story, increasingly it has become the whole story. Suggest to a nurse that she brings immense technical skill to her job, and her tendency is to tell a story that dismisses or devalues that skill. Add that she or he has medical knowledge, and the nurse may almost recoil in horror.

Nurses talk a great deal about holistic care, but the picture they paint depicts what I've come to think of as "halfistic" care—the half they are convinced doctors don't do or can't be bothered with. Nurses almost seem to denigrate the medical and technical. One gets the feeling that medical or technical work is a distasteful duty that doctors and the medical system force nurses to shoulder. Instead of linking caring, emotion, and relationship formation to other nursing activities, nurses today often separate them. Some focus so heavily on the "caring"—defined as emotional and relational work—that they ignore the medical and technical aspects of their work. More important, nurses may have become so focused on the relational that many neglect to mention that the nurse-patient relationship serves a set of instrumental goals—recovery, cure, coping, or perhaps a decent death. With the best of intentions, nurses seem devoted to convincing the public that nursing is more about friendship than about saving lives and preventing physical and emotional suffering.

The Rebellion against Cartesianism

In their 1989 book *The Primacy of Caring*, Patricia Benner and Judith Wrubel analyze the limitations of a reductionist, or Cartesian, view of the world. Benner and Wrubel explain that reductionists, who descend from the British empiricists—including philosopher John Locke—impose a mechanistic view on human life and experience. "For reductionists," they write, "the complex can best be understood in terms of its basic, atomic components, components that bear no intrinsic relation to one another."[2] Based on the philosophical tenets of the seventeenth-century French philosopher René Descartes, mechanistic thinking also argues that there is only one way to know human beings, through "representation." As the authors explain, Descartes insisted that "the mind and the body are distinct entities. In his view, the mind exists in time only, whereas the body, unlike the mind, is physical and has extension in space." The mind, which doesn't come in direct contact with the "external world," conjures "representations" that are "more or less correct approximations of reality. The contents of the mind are private, accessible only to the individual. Behavior by contrast is public and available for all to see."[3]

The authors thus explain that personal meanings, feelings, and "self-report" become suspect, and scientists—and by extension the public and policy community—come to depend only on objective data, which is not personal, emotionally tainted, or anecdotal. To be individual is to be "skewed," not to be trusted, and to be often dismissed. "Personal meanings are not only private but also a less than perfect apprehension of what is really out there in the world."[4] Benner and Wrubel propose that we replace the Cartesian view of the world with one that overcomes the "mind-body dualism"[5] of Cartesianism that has "dominated scientific thought for centuries." Benner and Wrubel propose a different, Heideggerian (after the German philosopher Martin Heidegger) way of thinking about the world that is phenomenological and that occurs when "the individual one stands outside the situation but is also involved in it."

For Benner and Wrubel the path to knowledge is through "embodied intelligence."[6] This includes "understanding the various rapid, nonexplicit, and nonconscious ways of grasping the significance of the situation for the self that are available for human beings." It involves what Benner and Wrubel call the "primacy of caring." This encompasses concern, solicitude, advocacy, and facilitation, which "empowers the Other to be what he or she wants to be, and this is the ultimate goal in nursing care relationships."[7]

As Benner moved on to describe "nurses' ways of knowing" and doing, she focused not only on the emotional ways they know the patient. In the many books and articles she has written with a variety of colleagues, her exemplars show nurses making medical diagnoses; teaching doctors about diseases and treatments; diagnosing subtle changes in patients' conditions; juggling complex medications, machines, and technologies; and dealing with the body as well as the soul. Although Benner has increasingly focused on the ethical nature of nurses' activities, the nurses she describes deal with the physical, the medical, and the technical.

When nurses began to talk about caring in the 1980s, theoreticians of "nurses' ways of knowing," such as Patricia Benner, clearly placed their discussions in a feminist context. This was an era of great feminist ferment, an era that produced such books as Jean Baker Miller's *Toward a New Psychology of Women*, Carol Gilligan's *In a Different Voice*, and Mary Field Belenky and her colleagues' book *Women's Way of Knowing*.[8] Like feminists outside of nursing, feminists in nursing were trying to give legitimacy to activities that had been long discounted in patriarchal society. It is interesting that what began as a kind of feminist revolt against patriarchy within nursing has led to what often reads like a reassertion of the kind of classical gender stereotypes that have long plagued the profession and women in general. Nurses, women, are associated with the soft and fluffy and doctors with the hard and scientific, as in nurses have hearts, while doctors have brains. In North America at least, the mantra has become that "doctors cure and nurses care," that, as nurses tell me over and over again, "doctors take care of diseases but nurses take care of the people who have them."

As caring discourse has evolved, it has been translated in academic programs and texts, in narratives that nurses prepare when they apply for clinical excellence awards and recruitment and retention campaigns. As individual nurses and nursing groups talk about their work, several important shifts have taken place. Nurses increasingly ignore the physical, medical, and technical, and when such aspects of care are mentioned, nurses tend to dismiss and devalue them or detach them from the emotional, psychosocial, and educational components of their job. Indeed, many nurses seem to voice an increasing disinterest in the body and in the hard work of physical care. Their work is often described almost entirely in terms of heart work. The fact that the brain guides their emotional labor is rarely acknowledged. They often belittle or render invisible the skill involved in the most emotional and relational of encounters. This may leave the listener or reader with the impression that nursing is feeling work based on female intuition, not intellectual work based on expert knowledge and experienced practice.

Ironically, this new nursing discourse is as mechanistic, reductionist, and incomplete as the one it was supposed to replace. Rather than presenting the embodied experiences that patients have, many nurses now talk about their work in a way that disembodies the patient. It also creates a reductionist view of the care of the sick in which different nursing activities "have no intrinsic relationship to one another." This disjuncture between their work and the way nurses talk about it introduces a new kind of dualism between mind and body. It almost seems as if there has become only one legitimate—or what Michel Foucault would have called "authoritative"—discourse in nursing. It is a discourse that severs the connection between talking the talk and walking the walk.

Devaluing the Medical and Technical Aspects of Nursing Work

In defining why and how their work makes a difference to patients, many nurses today dismiss, or sometimes even denigrate, the medical knowledge and technical skill they have amassed. I recently asked students in two American schools of nursing to write short anecdotes describing how their work makes a difference to patients. Some of the students were RNs with four-year degrees who were returning to school to get advanced practice degrees. I asked the students to use ordinary language to describe their work to a wider public. The majority described patients who had complex illnesses. Yet almost all of them ignored the physical, medical, or technical aspects of the care they must have provided these patients. Rather than combining their skills and knowledge into a concrete whole, they left their accounts full of holes by focusing exclusively on the psychosocial.

One ICU nurse, for example, described a patient who was HIV positive and had been admitted to her unit with *Pneumocystis carinii* pneumonia. Over the course of three pages, the RN describes how wonderful the patient was, how much he meant to her, and how she related to him. Her primary mission, according to the anecdote, was to show him "there was a familiar face and confidant when his direct family was unable to visit." She said that she "respected" her patient and learned from him. Although she saw this patient "from the time of his diagnosis till the time of his death," there is not a word about the physical care she delivered, the complex medications she administered, the technology and physiological processes she monitored. This patient had a long stay in the ICU. Yet she did not mention the role she played in preventing further infection, bedsores, deep vein thrombosis, pulmonary embolus, or urinary tract infection. Instead, we learn only about her psychological work with him:

> I learned that a nurse becomes the main support for her patient, and as well as treating them in the physical sense [something she does not describe], but more importantly, a nurse helps them to be comfortable in their illness and course of treatment. I had to use my nursing skills to help Mr. X be physically comfortable and I had to use my nurse judgments and psychology knowledge to help him feel comfortable with me, and feel like he could confide in me, and help him to deal with his fears.

Although highlighting the psychosocial and emotional certainly illuminates one aspect of nursing care, it does not require that the nurse downplay other areas of her work. When she reduces nursing practice to the provision of a familiar face, she may—albeit inadvertently—be helping pave the way for the RN to be replaced by a nurse's aide who can provide the same sense of familiarity at a much cheaper cost.

In another anecdote, a nurse describes taking care of a patient who has had a brain tumor for a year before his admission. She receives the patient on report and then describes the goals of her care. "Throughout my shift I assessed Mr. G.'s vital signs and changed his position, but those were the only physical interventions I performed during the shift." These physical interventions were, however, "not the client's most important need. The family and the client needed me to address their pain and I was able to alleviate some of their pain by using compassion, empathy, and open communication." Interestingly, she makes no mention of any physical pain the patient might have had and how she managed that complex activity. While this nurse talks about the emotional difficulty the family and patient experience because of the patient's worsening condition, she seems uninterested in or almost dismissive of the physical problems a patient like this encounters. She seems equally uninterested in the many medical and technical skills a nurse would mobilize in caring for this kind of patient.

This dichotomization of the medical and technical is nowhere more evident than in the following nurse's description of the essence of the role of the oncology nurse. As she writes about her work in a cancer center infusion unit, this particular oncology nurse talks about her work with a patient who just had a total abdominal hysterectomy after being diagnosed with ovarian cancer. To make sure the reader understands the role of the oncology nurse, she begins her anecdote by immediately defining what is—and is not—important about her role:

> People may think the most important part of being an oncology nurse is inserting an IV, accessing a port-a-catheter, administering antinausea medication, or infusing chemotherapy. This is not true. The part of my job that makes the greatest impact is educating patients to take care of oneself safely and efficiently at home. Providing patients with knowledge that they can comprehend and utilize in their daily life is what allows them to breathe easy and sleep at night. Oncology nurses help patients to maintain a good quality of life while being treated for cancer. A patient's well-being is dependent on the teaching they receive during chemotherapy treatment. Nursing is more than the tasks that are accomplished, it is all the roles one combines to give patients the power to care for themselves, physically, mentally, and emotionally.

This rendition of the role of the nurse is worth analyzing in some depth. The patient she goes on to describe has a potentially terminal illness. Ovarian cancer, after all, has a very high mortality rate. The patient has just had surgery, is in considerable pain, will be having chemotherapy—which this nurse will presumably deliver—and perhaps even radiation treatments. Rather than describing a total package of care—a package that includes the medical, technical, emotional, and even spiritual—the nurse divides and fragments and, ultimately devalues, one set of activities as she emphasizes the importance of another. The most important role of the nurse, she tells us, is educating the patient to take care of herself at home. Her role as a nurse is to support the patient and assure that she has quality of life while she is being treated for cancer. With her statement "This is not true," however, she sets up a sort of Berlin Wall between the medical and technical activities of her work and the educational and psychosocial.

But think about how the two sets of activities are, in fact, intrinsically interconnected. The nurse states that inserting an IV, accessing a port, managing nausea and vomiting, and infusing chemo are somehow less important than educating the patient. What would happen, however, if the activities this nurse seems to consider to be of second order importance are done incorrectly, without the skill and mastery of an experienced oncology nurse. If an IV is incorrectly inserted, toxic chemotherapy drugs may infiltrate the patient's skin and can, on rare occasions, burn it so badly that skin grafts may be necessary. If a port-a-catheter is not accessed with proper sterile technique, the patient may develop a serious, even fatal, blood infection. If the patient is vomiting uncontrollably, she can become dehydrated and malnourished and could require rehospitalization. If the patient develops other symptoms, such as stomatitis, mucositis, that are poorly managed, she may decide to forgo chemotherapy altogether. Finally, if the chemotherapy drugs are infused improperly, the medication will not attack the cancer cells.

If any of the above were to happen, the patient would have no quality of life and would not get to go home. There would thus be no opportunity for the nurse to educate her about how to "safely and efficiently" care for herself outside of the hospital setting. If any of the preventable complications described above occurred, the nurses caring for this patient would be so busy administering the medical and technical assistance she seems to devalue that they would have little opportunity to support the patient in other ways.

Imagine what could happen if a nurse looks down on these activities as less important than supporting and educating the patient. Can we have confidence that she will fully attend to the activities she seems to value so little? Study after study documents that patients value most the truly holistic caregiver—the one who combines caring with competence. Above all else, patients want a nurse who knows what she or he is doing from the medical and technical point of view. If that nurse is kind and compassionate then that is the perfect package. Yet, many contemporary nurses seem to devalue skills and activities their patients consider to be central. For example, one nursing student wrote about a woman with tongue cancer who had had two-thirds of her tongue removed. She had also had a tracheotomy tube and a g-tube inserted. Instead of holistically linking the physical body and terrible emotional burden the patient was bearing, the nurse spoke only of the patient's considerable emotional burden. "Aside from the fact that she was recovering from surgery," she reported, almost as if this were a minor detail, "she was lonely, scared, depressed, and grieving the loss of parts of her body and their functions. It was these issues that concerned me."

The Disappearance of the Body and the Denial of Nurses' Technical Expertise

In her excellent book *Devices and Desires: Gender, Technology, and American Nursing* Margarete Sandelowski explores the role nurses have played in the implementation of medical technology. From the introduction of the thermometer to the contemporary fetal monitor, Sandelowski documents how medicine depends on nursing for its reputation for scientific and technical mastery:

Nurses were and remain key components of the infrastructure of medical technology, yet they continue to retain the invisibility that all infrastructures, interfaces, and connecting links have. Nurses continue to be described as the glue or cement that holds the U.S. health care delivery system together, but like all glue and cement, they are not noticed in the overall structure.

The irony is that the very, often dramatic presence of devices, even those "spectacular" technologies that allowed clinicians new ways and new things to see, has not remedied the traditional cultural invisibility of nursing. New technologies have not so much resolved as dramatized the in-betweenness of the nurse. Indeed, as the quintessential boundary workers, regularly crossing the terrain between patient and physician, disease and illness, and medical and everyday practices, nurses have found and actively positioned themselves between patient and machine.[9]

Nurses actually save patients' lives. They know a lot about medical treatments and procedures. If they don't, they can't do their job. Their work involves the physical body as well as the patient's mind and spirit. But you would never know that from the way many nurses talk about their concrete daily practice, where their lifesaving manipulation of medical treatments and technologies is so often rendered invisible. In my sample, a pediatric burn nurse, for example, briefly mentions the need for sterile technique, infection control, and pain management in her work. Skittering past these details, she hastens to assure us that she is not too technically or medically oriented. To emphasize this fact, she zeroes in on the "harmful effects of burn trauma on the psyche," and the role nurses play in "emotional catharsis."

Why, one wonders, would it be a bad thing for the public to know how this nurse saves the patient's physical body? Do most members of the public recognize the lifesaving role burn nurses play in the care of the severely affected burn patients? Do many people realize that if the burn patients live long enough to have trouble coping with the trauma of a life after the burn unit, it's because of the complex physical care burn nurses give?

In her book, Sandelowski talks about the effect on nurses of the "in-between" role nurses play. To present this "in-betweenness"—this bridging role—nurses must depict the two shores they are connecting or various activities and perspectives they are bridging. In my analysis of nurses' stories, I have found that many fail to do this because they deliberately retreat from any mention of the medical and technical terrain. In fact, in a perfect illustration of the new Cartesianism, some adamantly reject any attempt to discuss the way they link medical, physical, and technical aspects of care with other aspects of their work.

As I have pondered why nurses seem to be so intent on concealing so many areas of their expertise, I've concluded that they are taught the skills of retreat in the subtle and not-so-subtle messages they receive in the course of their education and working lives. Many nurses in the academic field, for example, seem to highlight emotional caring and give it priority over other aspects of nursing activities. In so doing, they create a kind of grand narrative of care that overshadows the technical and medical. Nursing organizations also participate in the creation of a grand nursing narrative that rejects or conceals the full range of activities in which nurses engage.

This grand narrative is on exhibit when nursing organizations promote clinical excellence awards. To apply for such awards, nurses are often asked to write a clinical narrative or exemplar describing their work with a particular patient. The American Association of Critical Care Nurses (AACCN), one of the largest professional nursing organizations, has, for example, created Circle of Excellence awards. Nurses are provided with an elaborate instruction brochure that counsels them on how to apply for these awards. To be eligible, members must submit an exemplar that shows, "where, in your opinion, your intervention really made a difference in a patient's outcome." For its year 2000 awards, the AACCN brochure included a sample of a winning exemplar by Beverly D'Angio, who described her relationship with a young child with a "complex congenital heart disease" who was treated on her pediatric ICU.[10]

The boy, named Brandon, was waiting for a new heart. In a two-page, fifteen-paragraph exemplar, D'Angio chronicles the boy's deterioration and his ultimate death. Although there is the occasional mention of a medical or technical detail—"He began to develop additional dysrhythmias and severe metabolic acidosis"—the nurse's account does not address how she dealt with this problem or any of the medical or technical issues she would presumably have addressed over the course of his hospital stay. Instead, her nursing interventions include worrying about the boy, fearing for his fate, commiserating with other members of the health care team, such as pastoral care workers, and talking with his anguished parents. Taking the oft repeated injunction of nurse educators to heart, D'Angio has placed herself so totally "on the same level" as the patient and family that she becomes indistinguishable as a professional or clinician. Rather than discussing the multiple ways in which her professional knowledge and action made a difference to her patient and his family, she talks about the anguish she felt, the many hugs she distributed, how much she cried when he died, and how strongly she bonded with his family. In this entirely sentimentalized account, she writes about seeing the patient's mother in the hospital after he dies. "The first time I saw her in the hall, we hugged and cried," she writes.

This account is important because with the best of intentions a large nursing organization considered it to be an excellent example of the nurses' holistic approach and presented it as a storytelling guide for other nurses who were constructing their own narratives of care. Indeed, no matter where nurses work or study, they seem to shape their definitions of their work around this basic template and resist altering it. About a year ago, for example, I talked with nurse-practitioner students in a well-respected program in the Northeast. The class included experienced RNs going back to school to get their NP degree and people with a four-year degree in another subject but no nursing background, who were being fast-tracked into NP work. When I asked the students to describe the work of the NP, all of them talked about the "holistic" approach of the nurse-practitioner. In their discussion of "holism," they focused exclusively on psychosocial and emotional aspects of care. When I asked them about their medical knowledge of diseases and drugs they seemed almost angry. "We take a holistic approach," one reiterated. When I suggested that holism includes the medical, she became distressed, insisting over and over again on "holism." Baffled by this response, I asked, "Doesn't holism include knowledge of routine medical conditions and your ability to diagnose them as well as to prescribe routine medical treatments? After all, don't nurse-practitioners differ from the bedside nurse because they are legally permitted to diagnose routine conditions and prescribe medications? Wouldn't it be good to mention that?" I suggested.

Apparently not. This particular student felt that any mention of the medical would take away from the "nursing approach" and compromise the claim to holism. Another nurse, already an RN, agreed. She seemed distraught by the idea that nurses would want to advertise their medical knowledge. To do so, she insisted, would be to "downplay" the holistic or psychosocial. Although I repeatedly insisted that I wanted the students to combine—not counterpose—it seemed difficult for them to capture that concept. "We have been trying to define our work with no success ever since I have been in nursing," the RN said in an agitated tone. "Trying to find something that is our own, that no one can take away from us. Finally, we have it. The NP role. We are the patient's partner, we give holistic care. We are patient-centered. And you are trying to take that away from us."

When I was in Switzerland in 2005, several professors of nursing made the same argument. "If we do what you suggest, we risk losing everything, everything," one professor at a well-known nursing school said, shaking her head somberly. "You know doctors are so powerful here."

The idea that talking about the medical, technical, or physical aspects of the nurses role is "trying to take something away from" the nurse or profession is deep-seated. When Sioban Nelson and I discuss the impact of the virtue script in nursing and on the public image of the nurse, many nurses interpret this as denigrating caring and arguing for its opposite. Some see any effort to move beyond a sentimentalized caring script as being unwise, even dangerous, for nursing. As one young nurse once told me, "The public trusts us because we are so caring. If we talk about other things we will lose public trust."

It would be hard to imagine a physician saying something analogous. Most doctors would feel perfectly comfortable explaining that they have attained great technical skill and have extensive experience in diagnosing and treating a particular condition. They trumpet the fact that they have degrees or experience in other fields—for example, in public health, anthropology, or history. Numerous physicians advertise their work as poets, novelists, or essayists. Most important, they are thrilled to claim that they are also aces at caring. Physicians would claim it all and would understand that, in making that claim, public trust would be enhanced not diminished.

In our chapter on the virtue script in nursing, Nelson and I ask why the language of traditional feminine virtues is so appealing and pervasive within nursing. This is surprising, we argue, because so many other professional women have tried to move beyond the traditional image of the good woman doing good works to show the knowledge work involved in their professional practice. One can ask the same question here: Why are nurses so intent on concealing their medical knowledge and technical skills and so determined to escape the physical bodies to which they are, through their work, so clearly attached?

One reason nurses may be intent on unlinking mind and body may have to do with their desire to escape the "tasks" to which they feel they are tethered by medicine, technology, and the patient's relentless physical needs. This retreat from "tasks" is an understandable reaction against nursing's long association with performance of a series of disaggregated, so-called mindless activities that are accorded low status in the medical system. As I explained in my book *Nursing against the Odds*, in the nineteenth century the medical profession determined to reduce nursing work to the performance of a series of mindless activities.[11] The minds behind both medical and nursing care belonged to physicians, not nurses, and in the early twentieth century this led sociologists to assign nursing to the social purgatory of being a "semi-profession."[12] This definition has haunted nurses to this day, and many believe that the tasks have turned would-be professionals into "just nurses." In order to escape this categorization, many nurses routinely insist that nursing is not a collection of "tasks" but rather the application of "critical thinking skills" and "judgment" to patient problems.

Although this response it understandable, it is a professional-legiti-mating strategy of limited utility. Rather than illuminating the education and skill that is required to do tasks that have been deemed to be mindless, many nurses avoid talking about the concrete, routine daily activities in-volved in their work. After all, a doctor could delegate a nursing task to me—a very highly educated person, although not in nursing—and I would be utterly unable to implement it.

Because, as Sandelowski puts it, nurses themselves have "inadvertently complied with the prevailing cultural practice of denigrating the very 'body knowledge' that is the forte of the nurse," nursing becomes, in some academic discourse, almost unknowable.[13] If their professors and organiza-tional "leaders" devalue the tasks involved in nursing, then the nurses who perform those tasks will get very little encouragement to talk about them in ways that illuminate what they are doing and why they are doing it.

Sandelowski's discussion of this caring/curing dichotomy is helpful:

> While nurses at the bedside turned to technology largely to improve their care and their status, academically oriented nurses eager to undermine the image of the nurse as merely a doer and nursing as a set of procedures began to turn away from technology after World War II. Theories of nursing that emerged in the 1950s and 1960s etherealized, disembodied, and dema-terialized nursing in order to emphasize the minds, as opposed to the hands, of nurses. The "discourse on caring" that emerged in the 1980s, with its explicitly anti-technology bias, was itself a "technology of gender (and) morality" that academic nurses used to revalorize the feminine in nursing. These nurses used language as a technology to construct nursing as beyond or as frankly opposed to technology.[14]

The parlous state of contemporary nurse and physician relationships doesn't help matters. Many nurses will studiously avoid talking about the medical aspects of their work because they perceive the "medical" to be what the doctor has ordered. Thus, when the oncology nurse downplayed the importance of "medical" aspects of chemotherapy administration, she may have done so because she associates those activities with what a doctor has ordered her to do. Either in her formal or in the informal nursing cur-riculum, she may have been taught to avoid discussing these activities be cause to do so would be to focus on what is distinctly "medicine's domain," not that of nursing.

Obviously, not every doctor's treatment recommendation is appropriate. In this case, however, that wasn't the issue. To retreat from what is per-ceived to be the "medical" or the doctor's orders places the nurse in a para-doxical situation. The vast majority of a cancer nurse's time is spent in administering and monitoring cancer treatment. If a cancer nurse does not want to be involved in and refuses to claim the central importance of her role in cancer treatment, she will be limiting both public understanding of her work and her ability to claim a legitimate role in the health care system.

When nurses disclaim their own considerable medical expertise this also ratifies the erroneous notion that only doctors have medical knowledge, make medical judgments, and take medical actions. To so discount their contributions in these areas allows members of the public to believe that doctors function "autonomously." If nurses were, on the other hand, to claim credit for their contributions to activities that we believe to be exclusively medical, this would help us all understand that physicians, like other clinicians, function in a web of clinical relationships. Many other clinicians play a critical role in what we imagine to be the doctor's sole domain—diagnosis, treatment and prescription, and technological and scientific mastery. When nurses focus only on nursing knowledge, nursing diagnosis, education and caring, they depict themselves as the ones who do the bits the doctors don't want to do.

Implications

One of the most serious problems of the new Cartesianism in nurses' storytelling is that nurses cede to doctors the cures that they, as nurses, advance. Traditional dichotomies thus persist and are reinforced: doctors do the big things, nurses do little things; doctors do visible things, nurses do invisible things; doctors use science and data, nurses use intuition. Doctors are sung heroes, but, as the recent Johnson & Johnson Campaign for Nursing's Future jingle puts it, nurses are unsung heroes, content, for their reward, with the gratitude in a patient's eyes.[15] Or, as a British image campaign describes it, nurses have "quiet power," while doctors, by implication, are the noisy ones.[16] Indeed, so deeply entrenched are these stereotypes that it sometimes seems as if being overlooked were somehow a badge of honor. One sometimes feels that nurses are, in this way, asserting a kind of moral superiority over doctors, who are not only depicted as money grubbing but as publicity and recognition hogs as well. If this is the moral frame of reference, it's understandable that nurses would do little to illuminate how they participate in those activities commonly considered to be the exclusive province of medicine. If caring is their claim to the moral high ground, it is understandable that nurses would be quite happy to remain in their own cordoned- off territory of the relational, caring, and psychosocial.

Perhaps the most serious problem with this contemporary Cartesianism is that it misconstrues the nature and purpose of the kind of relational work nurses do. Over and over again, nurses describe the essence of their work as "relational." Although nurses constantly emphasize this relational aspect of nursing, many seem to profoundly misunderstand how relationships with patients are formed and what ends these relationships serve. When I watched nurses for three years at Boston's Beth Israel Hospital, it became clear to me that nurses were able to form relationships with patients because they were constantly doing for and with patients. They were giving them bed-baths, helping them to the toilet, administering their medications, observing how they reacted to their treatments, helping them to eat or walk, changing their dressings, debriding their wounds, yes, even cleaning up their vomit, urine, and feces. Throughout all of these physically and medically based encounters, the nurse talked and listened to her patient, discovering, in the process, how her patient responded to illness and its treatment, not only physically and medically but emotionally and sometimes even spiritually. Nurses could claim a holistic understanding of the patient because they delivered a broad spectrum of care and engaged in a wide spectrum of activities that made up the whole. They elicited the patient's experience of illness as it was lived across the trajectory of illness and disease and dysfunction.

The nurse-patient relationship emerged from and was forged through the physical, domestic, educational, teaching, talking, walking experiences the nurse had with her patient. Unlike a psychotherapist or social worker, relationships in the nursing of the sick and vulnerable did not arise because a patient consulted a clinician so that he or she could recount and analyze their problems. With the exception of the nurse who is a specialist in psychiatry or psychotherapy, most nurses involved in the direct care of sick patients form relationships that are an outgrowth of the physical, medical, and technical care that the nurse provides the patient.

As I observed these relationships being formed, I understood that they depended on the provision of bodily care that gave the nurse intimate, immediate, urgent contact with the patient, often over a long period of time. The medical, technical, and physical was not ancillary to relationship but intrinsically connected to it, because it is the provision of that care that gives the nurse access and connection to a patient. It is through that kind of caregiving that he or she is able to gather the kind of critical information about the patient on which relationship depends.

Which brings me to the second point about the nurse-patient relationship, or the relational work, that is at the heart of nursing. The trust established between patient and nurse is not only built because it links the nurse and patient in a humanistic relationship. It is also instrumental because it helps that nurse find out critical things about the patient, both physical and emotional. Is the patient taking her medication? Why not? Do they understand it has to be taken with food? Three times a day, not once? For ten days, not two? Is the patient so afraid of the surgery that his blood pressure will shoot up? What can help calm him down? Why does the patient want to discontinue the chemotherapy that may give her a remission from breast cancer? Is it because, as was true in a case I described in *Life Support*, her husband is beating her and her children are uncontrollable?[17] What can be done to deal with her problems and save her life? Is a patient walking after surgery? Why not? How can he be helped to do so and thus saved from the risk of deep vein thrombosis and a pulmonary embolism? Has the patient had it with chemotherapy and would she prefer to give up the fight and die?

Patients need nurses because nurses are the ones who save their lives, prevent mistakes and complications, and do so in a way that recognizes that there is a human being who is being assaulted by a particular disease or disorder. For most patients, nursing care is not about the provision of friendship. Most people aren't admitted to the hospital because they have a friendship disorder—and if they are, then they need another kind of clinician–a psychiatrist, or psychiatric nurse or social worker.

Of course, there are times when patients want the nurse to be there to accompany them through their suffering and their journey. But I believe a patient will ask this of a nurse precisely because the nurse has done things with and for the patient. It is through the provision of competent, humane care that the nurse becomes someone the patient trusts to witness her suffering or to whom she can confide her dilemmas. It is because the nurse has done things with or to the patient that the patient may want her to stop doing and start being. And, as the work of palliative care nurses demonstrates, even that "being with" is a skilled activity.

Yet, today, listening to nurses and nursing students talk about their work, it seems almost as if the nurse-patient relationship exists solely for the sake of the relationship. It often appears that this relationship has no instrumental component and is not built in the service of cure, recovery, remission, coping, or even a decent death. Sometimes the focus on relationship, as some nurses describe it, seems to be less about the patient and more about the nurse and the difference the patient made to her. Again, this kind of response does not play well to administrators, journalists, or policymakers eager to contain health care costs. We don't pay nurses so patients can make a difference to them or so that they can be purveyors of social justice or spiritual guides. We pay them to make a difference to patients and patient outcomes.

Although I understand the complex constellation of factors that encourages nurses to construct their work in the ways I have described, this new Cartesian construction of nursing is dangerous for a number of reasons. First and foremost it is simply not an accurate picture of what most nurses do and certainly does not encompass what most patients want—and what they desperately need—from nurses. Because it so poorly captures nurses' work, using this kind of descriptive language to argue for the presence of nurses at the bedside, in the clinic, hospice, rehab hospital, or wherever sick people need nursing care is a recipe for disaster. When hospitals post job descriptions they do not usually advertise for hospital humanists, as one hospital administrator who was very pro-nursing but equally frustrated with nursing rhetoric, recently told me. Enhance patient outcomes, save money, deliver needed care, prove that compassion counts because it helps you better deliver that care, and you have a chance. Focus only on the relational and humanistic, as Dana Beth Weinberg explains, and you have little chance of convincing bottom-line-oriented administrators and elected officials that you play a critical life and cost-saving role in the health care system.

Linked to this, if nurses do not value the physical, the embodied, the medical, and technical, how can they attend to it? Even if they do not, themselves, provide that direct care to patients, how can we trust that they will appropriately manage or relate to those nurses or nursing assistants that do? If people overlook this kind of activity in their descriptions of their work, how can we be assured that they will not overlook it in their practice? And if they do, how can they practice holistically and protect their patients from the myriad risks that illness and infirmity entail?

When I recently spoke at a nursing conference in Australia, Barry Morley, a critical care nurse in a Perth hospital, asked me an interesting question. When patients express concerns about nursing care to hospital management, their complaints spotlight the nurse who didn't have time to hold their hand or give them a back rub. They never write in to complain because we didn't have time to prevent a complication or engage in some other lifesaving activity. Why is that? he asked.

It's probably because people, like my lawyer friend and the journalists who interviewed me on radio and TV, don't really understand the lifesaving work that nurses do. Is that because, as so many nurses insist, doctors, the media, and even hospital administrators have made their work invisible? Or is it because modern nursing discourse is, with all the best of intentions, keeping it invisible? Or both?

8

Nurses Must Be Clever to Care

Sanchia Aranda and Rosie Brown

Are nurses "too clever to care" these days? Some commentators certainly think so. The headline from the April 25, 2004, edition of the London *Sunday Times* raised the question, when reporting on a resolution debated at the 2004 congress of the Royal College of Nursing. According to the media reports, this proposal declared "nurses are too clever to care." The delegates heard the argument that nurses should no longer undertake tasks such as the provision of hygiene and other essential body care functions often referred to as "basic nursing care," with many delegates drawing a clear distinction between the technical and caring aspects of nursing. One striking aspect of the debate was that although nurses were able to describe these technical aspects as tasks such as cannulation, the language they mobilized to describe caring was seriously impoverished. Some nurses seemed to assume that the words care and caring had universal meaning and inherent importance. Others referred to vague notions of holism or simply equated caring with assistance in hygiene. One speaker even described caring as the privilege of carrying the excreta of his patient. Ninety-five percent of the congress delegates voted to defeat the resolution, thus asserting that clever nurses are indeed needed to care. Nonetheless, the debate signals an important development inside nursing that merits serious consideration.

To the public nursing is often associated with distasteful tasks such as handling excreta. There is very little public understanding of the knowledge base of nursing practice. This is hardly surprising since nurses themselves often struggle to articulate the skill and knowledge at the center of caring practices, and many may not even value it. The *Sunday Times* head-line, "Nurses Are Too Clever to Care for You," implies that knowledge work in nursing is only involved in those dimensions of practice that are not associated with care of the person, or more narrowly with the person's body. Thus, the care of the body is understood as natural and unskilled (often abstract and elusive) while technical practices are skilled and based on knowledge (definable and precise).

In this chapter we critique the dismissal of "basic nursing care" as a nonessential component of nursing knowledge and practice activity. Such care is critical to both the delivery of expert nursing and to any under-standing of nurses' contribution to health care. We will draw on studies from the past decade of nurses in cancer and palliative care settings.[1] These studies illuminated the expertise present in everyday practice, an expertise largely invisible in the everyday language of nursing. They raise significant concerns about the substantial shift in nursing away from "basic nursing care" and the promotion of roles considered "advanced practice," in which the nurse engages in less direct patient care and acts as a consultant or ad-viser to others. These roles tend to leave basic nursing care to the least qual-ified worker and emphasize or give priority to the talking and psychosocial dimensions of care. This results in nursing work and the work of caring it-self becoming bifurcated and increasingly defined as either "doing" or "talking," with the latter seen as more skilled and of higher status.

Caring as interpersonal, relational work has become the primary way nurses and nursing understand caring as a central nursing activity. This focus has led to a decreasing emphasis on the importance of caring as doing or delivering basic nursing care. Using the example of palliative care we suggest that moving skilled and knowledgeable nurses away from body work, through, for example, the creation of "case management" roles, may lead to increased status for the nurse but result in fragmented and inferior care for patients. At its extreme this fragmentation may make the nurse un-able to see the extent to which the patient's needs remain unmet. This can happen when "basic nursing care" is abandoned to less skilled workers or limits are imposed in the care systems nurses work in but fail to success-fully challenge.

As nursing moves into the twenty-first century, the dominant under-standing of nursing work by the public, and within the profession, is that nursing is primarily the delivery of interpersonal care. In great part this is fueled by efforts at cost-cutting and market models imposed on hospitals and health care systems. In an attempt to deliver nursing care more cheaply, institutions try to substitute cheaper workers for more expensive, more skilled workers. In this construction of care many core dimensions that make up complex nursing practice are left out of the picture and discussion. As a result, systems of care, often driven by these economic imperatives, may be supported by nurses trying to adapt to contemporary conditions. As this occurs, both economic models and nurses' adaptation to them are changing the roles of nurses in ways that emphasize nonbody aspects of work, particularly interpersonal caring. Thus, in practice the work of the most educated nurses is becoming less concerned with care of the patient's body. This kind of care is increasingly left to cheaper unskilled workers. The increasing separation between doing and talking work risks fragmenting the care sick patients receive. As nursing roles become more narrowly defined this may lead to a deskilling of the nursing workforce. What will be lost is attention to the complex interplay between the patient, his or her disease, and the physical and psychosocial consequences of being sick.

We suggest that the dominance of interpersonal care in nursing and its being given priority over basic nursing care has unintended but negative consequences for both patients and the profession. Using examples of nursing work, we argue that current conceptualizations of caring deemphasize the skilled work inherent in basic nursing care; place greater importance on interpersonal care at the expense of basic nursing care as the primary work of nurses; sanitize (by making it invisible) the skilled work of nurses caring for people with diseased bodies; and fail to capture the complex interplay between physical, technical, and interpersonal caring that lies at the heart of skilled nursing practice.

The Rise of Caring in Nursing

An examination of contemporary nursing literature might suggest that caring in nursing has always been concerned with the interpersonal relationship between nurse and patient. However, this is far from the case. Florence Nightingale, in her book *Notes on Nursing*, made observation central to the nursing role, which was to be the eyes and ears of the doctor.[2] She warned against the development of interpersonal relationships between nurses and patients. At the turn of the twentieth century writing about nursing was dominated by medical interests. The patient was understood as an object of interest to the doctor who sought to diagnose and treat disease. Nurses were engaged in servant-master relationships with doctors[3] and were increasingly understood as important to the doctor in the medical surveillance of the body.[4]

Traditionally, the focus of nurses' surveillance was the biological body. Nurses were expected to observe biological changes and report these to the doctor for potential intervention. Indeed, even today distinctions between the diagnostic role of nursing and medicine cast the nurse as an observer who passes on the information to the knowledgeable doctor. He then is able to make a diagnosis and prescribe treatment, which many members of the public wrongly believe the doctor administers.

Nursing has constantly tried to separate itself from medicine and to gain broader public recognition for nursing as a profession in its own right. By the 1950s nursing scholars, therefore, began to write about a unique body of knowledge that belonged to nursing. Although nurses' provision of medical treatments was a core part of nursing, it was portrayed as part of an interdependent rather than independent body of knowledge. The extent of this struggle for professional independence from medicine was evident in the explosion of efforts to develop nursing theory through the 1960s and 1970s. These produced theoretical perspectives as diverse as Dorothea Orem's self-care deficit model, which emphasized the nurse's role in compensating for functional deficits, to Rosemary Parse's theory of "Man-Living-Health," which explored the psychosocial domains of nursing and nurses' contribution to human existential growth.[5] Nursing theorists sought to resist the view that nursing existed simply to carry out the instructions of the doctor or to undertake the distasteful tasks that arise when bodies are diseased. These early theorists attempted to put into words the complex reality of nursing practice. Each resultant theory, although useful in understanding nursing in part, failed to capture the whole. One outcome of this theoretical work was the establishment of "caring" as the professional base of nursing. Nursing theorists juxtaposed the caring focus of nursing with the "curing" focus of medicine, often singling out and awarding priority to care over cure—a separation we are sure the public does not expect or support.

Caring was thus constructed as a framework that would liberate nurses from the dominance of scientific and medical perspectives in health care. Through this framework doctors were seen to be specifically concerned with the diseased body while nurses were concerned with the whole person. This theoretical work in nursing resulted in a metanarrative of caring constructed around theories that privileged and centralized interpersonal interactions in nursing. In most instances, caring, in a nursing sense, is premised on the relationship that is established between a nurse and a patient. Indeed, Jean Watson, an influential nurse theorist, argued that caring could only be demonstrated and practiced interpersonally; namely, in the context of a relationship that is established between the nurse and the patient.[6] Such perspectives take little account of nursing in situations where relationships cannot be formed such as in trauma care, when the person is unconscious or in so much pain that they simply cannot relate. Nor do they take into account the patient's primary desire to have someone deal competently with his or her diseased body.

This emphasis on the interpersonal dimensions of caring in nursing arose during the 1960s.[7] It was strongly influenced by the growing interest in personal psychology and communication. Before this, commentators suggested that a personal relationship between nurse and patient would be problematic in that it would bring feelings into the delivery of medical care and would thus increase the potential for anxiety in the nurse.[8] Isabel Menzies argued that the structure of nursing work sought to limit the development of interpersonal interaction in an effort to reduce this anxiety both for the individual nurse and for the organization.[9] The influence of theories of interpersonal caring on nursing was to expand the scope of nursing from provision of physical care and surveillance of the diseased body to work that took account of the patient's feelings and experiences. Nurses were thus encouraged to "know" the patient[10] and to understand not just the patient's physical experience but how they responded emotionally to disease and dysfunction.[11]

This changing nature of the nurse-patient relationship also resulted in a theoretical repositioning of what constitutes a good nurse. Relationship-centered care has become the new paradigm for nursing and health care.[12] A distant and impersonal nurse, albeit one with great technical efficiency and who appears unaffected by the suffering of those around her, is being replaced by "a nurse who is self-aware, able to cope with self-disclosure and with highly developed interpersonal skills."[13] The nurse's potential to help the patient is linked to the relationship between them, with the relationship given therapeutic potential.[14] Cool efficiency is being replaced by calls for the nurse to develop intimate, empathetic, and reciprocal relationships with patients, to be equal to or on the same level as the patient.

This theoretical work in nursing resulted in a metanarrative of caring constructed around theories that made interpersonal interactions central to nursing. However, before exploring this let us consider the nursing skill in basic nursing care, a body of knowledge that is underemphasized in the theoretical work on caring.

The Skilled Work Inherent in Basic Nursing Care

To illustrate the importance of basic nursing care we draw on the observational study of community palliative care nurses we did along with Judith Parker.[15] As part of a research degree in nursing, Brown observed over seventy interactions between nurses and people receiving care from a community palliative care program. A palliative care service was chosen because people who are dying experience bodily deterioration as their bodies decline and ultimately fail. This deterioration leads to physical symptoms such as pain, nausea, and tiredness, which in turn produce a loss of functional capacity and, commonly, a dependence on others for activities such as toileting and hygiene.

Our premise was that while suffering can be both physical and psychological, many of the issues causing psychological suffering are the end point of physical deterioration. It is this physical decline that alters the person's capacity to be in the world in ways that are meaningful to them. Examples include the mother who is now too frail to carry her infant child, the husband who can no longer be the breadwinner for his family, and the sports star who can no longer walk. Drawing from the work of Jocalyn Lawler[16] the aim of this study was to give voice to these poorly articulated aspects of skilled work in nursing in a practice setting (home care) where the only ones who often observe nursing work are patients and family members. This complex work is largely hidden even from other nurses, clinicians, and health care workers. Although they often struggled to clearly define this work, the nurses in this community palliative care service were able to describe the importance of "hands-on" care in their work.

In Australia, as in many other parts of the world, demands for access to specialist palliative care have resulted in nursing role changes. One of the most significant changes is a reduction in the amount of physical care specialist palliative care nurses perform as they embrace consultation and case management roles. These roles, in turn, support the work of less expensive generalist nurses and care assistants (and family carers) who provide most of the basic nursing care for patients at home. The rationale for this change in models of service delivery, while not formally documented, appears to be to ensure that access to the limited availability of specialist palliative care is made available to all those who need it. Government policies support increased access to specialist services but seek to achieve this through service sharing with generalist nursing services rather than through an increase in the availability of specialist services. The result is a rationing of specialist services and a substantial reduction in the amount of direct care specialist nurses give to patients. Instead, the specialist becomes increasingly focused on providing her expertise and support to nurses and nurse's aides who provide the direct care. Although patients do have access to specialist care, the specialist nurse is spread across more patients. The potential problems are illustrated when we examine the provision of direct care in this setting.

Consider, for example, a case that illustrates the importance of toileting in the care of an elderly Italian man with a primary malignant brain tumor.

Mr. C. was being cared for at home by his wife. A generalist community nursing service provided the couple with basic nursing care, which was supplemented by specialist palliative care staff who served as case managers. The specialist nurse provided direct input when needed for symptom management and psychosocial support. As Mr. C.'s condition deteriorated so did his English skills, making it difficult for nurses and aides to communicate with him. Researcher Brown sat in on an interview that the specialist palliative care nurse held with Mr. and Mrs. C. Because Mr. C. had such difficulty with English, the nurse predominantly interacted with Mrs. C. The two discussed critical issues such as changes in Mr. C.'s physical and mental status, medication requirements, and care needs, including those that surfaced during his recent periods of incontinence.

While Mrs. C. was out shopping that morning, Mr. C. had been incontinent. During the interview Mr. C. became restless. Brown and the specialist nurse recognized this as a signal that he had to go to the toilet. Brown volunteered to take Mr. C. to the bathroom. It would allow the nurse to continue her discussion with Mrs. C., and it would give her some important information about Mr. C.'s condition.

As she accompanied the old man to the bathroom, Brown noted how much critical information she gained through this seemingly minor task of physical assistance:

- Mr. C.'s restlessness was indeed due to the fact that he needed to go to the toilet. His subsequent relief suggested that he remained aware of the bodily signals for toileting.
- Mr. C. required assistance to walk. His gait was unbalanced and he appeared to have difficulty seeing. Whoever helped him to the toilet—nurse, aide, or wife—would need to support him and direct him to the bathroom.
- He had difficulty getting safely into and out of the bathroom and needed to be told where to stand and what hand rails to use.
- He needed assistance to get his pajama pants up and down.
- He needed direction and help in washing and drying his hands.

This information was not gained as part of a formal assessment in which the specialist nurse asked either the patient or his wife a particular set of questions. Indeed, because of Mr. C.'s difficulty with English in particular and communication in general, it could not have been gained in such an interview. Brown was able to discover Mr. C.'s needs because she saw them when she was taking him to the toilet. Yet the opportunity to gain this kind of knowledge is increasingly limited as such tasks are given to less skilled and knowledgeable nurses or aides.

From the information Brown gained and shared with the palliative care nurse they determined that the increase in Mr. C.'s incontinence was likely related to a functional inability to go to the toilet independently. These insights resulted in a different set of nursing interventions than would have occurred if the incontinence resulted from loss of control over bladder function, which might be managed by the use of condom drainage or even catheterization. Mr. C. retained bladder control but had lost the functional ability to respond to bladder signals. Nursing interventions included helping Mrs. C. to plan a regular toileting regimen for Mr. C. Other options might include providing a commode near Mr. C.'s chair or bedside so he could get to the toilet more easily.

The information also provided considerable insight into the burden Mrs. C. shouldered in caring for her husband. The couple would need increased support if Mr. C. was to remain at home. The specialist palliative care nurse could now address these significant changes in Mr. C.'s condition. The information helped her prepare for the couple's needs and create a supportive environment that recognized the interplay between the distress of watching someone you love die and the daily tangible reminders of death that accompany bodily decline. If such basic care was not a part of the specialist nurse's role the resultant plan of care for Mr. C. and support for Mrs. C. would have been considerably less effective and meaningful.

Splitting care between the specialist nurse providing support and the general community nurse providing physical care creates significant problems. The two nurses rarely visit the home together; they are in different workplaces, and thus have little opportunity for informal discussion about clinical care issues. Although some argue that important information can be gained in a formal assessment of functional capacity, the provision of basic care tasks such as toileting, and the information gleaned during them, provides information not easily gained in such assessments. An effective and comprehensive plan of care is more meaningful to the recipients when such information becomes part of the assessment. Indeed, this separation between support and direct care may be producing a cadre of new nurses that lack this skill and are thus deskilled at such integration. Although routine physical and psychosocial assessment is part of the basic education requirements for nurses, new graduates quickly find such skills receive little attention in practice in most settings.

Privileging Interpersonal Caring

Why has interpersonal caring displaced bodily care? This may be because of nurses' increasing knowledge of psychology and the role this plays in nurses' attempts to gain social legitimacy. When nurses began to include in their studies and research knowledge from personal psychology this gave the professional a powerful point of separation from medicine. The knowledge work associated with psychology transformed nursing into interpersonal caring, set nurses apart from medicine, and provided a legitimate platform on which to base knowledge development. However, this also set the stage for a disjunction between knowledge and practice at the practical level where nurses continue to be involved in the provision of basic nursing care to diseased bodies. In their descriptions and discussions of what is and is not important in nursing, interpersonal caring and psychosocial issues are seen as more skilled and therefore more important than understanding the physical (and disease-based) deterioration leading to the need for basic nursing care. The following example from Brown's study illustrates the temptation to give precedence to the interpersonal aspects of care over physical care.

Brown was observing a specialist palliative care nurse who was working with Mrs. S., a fifty-seven-year-old woman with lung cancer, which had spread to her bones and brain. The brain metastasis was causing considerable problems with mobility. Nurse Katherine Bower's[17] role as case manager placed emphasis on care coordination and psychological support for Mrs. S. and her husband, with her physical care needs met by the generalist home nursing service. An occupational therapist involved in Mrs. S.'s care had asked Nurse Bower to obtain a hospital bed for Mrs. S. so she could safely get in and out of bed. On the way to the visit, Nurse Bower told Brown that she was worried about the decision to bring in a hospital bed when Mrs. S. was still reasonably well. Although she had not discussed this with Mr. and Mrs. S., Nurse Bower believed this move could have a negative affect on the marital relationship and be interpreted as a signal of deterioration and approaching death.

Brown watched Nurse Bower as she asked the couple about their concerns. The couple said they were concerned about Mrs. S.'s increasing limb weakness and lack of mobility, which had resulted in a recent fall. A previous fall had caused a pathological fracture of Mrs. S.'s upper arm and the bone metastases meant that future fractures were likely if falls continued. Neither husband nor wife mentioned the need for a hospital bed. During the visit Nurse Bower was able to provide the couple with information about Mrs. S.'s deteriorating condition, convey relevant factual information, and sensitively explain that her deterioration and symptoms were unlikely to benefit from further medical intervention. She thus displayed the skilled nursing care that creates an environment to exchange information and raise sensitive issues that are critical in helping people adjust to a terminal illness. Nurse Bower did not, however, raise the issues the occupational therapist was concerned about, nor did she try to assess Mrs. S.'s mobility. She did not, for example, try to find out whether Mrs. S. had difficulty getting in and out of bed or whether the couple shared her concern about moving out of the marital and into a hospital bed.

The splitting of nursing into a specialist consulting or case management role (talking and psychosocial care) and a role in providing assistance with physical care (doing care) fragments the care the nurse delivers and deprives the patient of much-needed assistance and understanding. Imagine for a moment that Nurse Bower's role had included assisting Mrs. S. to shower. As she did this, the nurse would have observed Mrs. S. walk between bedroom and bathroom. She would have seen how Mrs. S. got into and out of the bed, which would have helped her determine whether Mrs. S. might benefit from aids that would help her get in and out of bed, such as an over-bed pulley, that might delay any need for a hospital bed. As she washed Mrs. S. she could provide useful safety hints such as how to move and turn using handrails or the use of walking aids. Mrs. S.'s husband could have been included in this discussion, helping him to carry out such tasks when the nurse was absent. This information and the activity of showering would have opened up opportunities to ask specific questions about Mrs. S.'s difficulty with mobility. Nurse Bower could have voiced her own concerns about the marital consequences of changing beds.

Specialist palliative care nurses claim more knowledge and expertise than generalist community nurses or aides. Nurse Bower could, therefore, combine precise assessment of Mrs. S.'s function with her knowledge of the progression of cancer and the likely symptoms and physical difficulties this would bring as her disease progressed.

Although Nurse Bower could certainly gain some information and understanding of Mrs. S.'s care requirements through a formal assessment (using predominantly verbal information and then combining it with formal knowledge and previous experience of similar patients), its effect on care provision would be lessened if it was not combined with insight into the specific needs and experiences of this particular patient. Formal assessments are crucial to the formal role of the nurse but are unlikely to lead to the disclosures of information critical to the ongoing care of patients. Much of what nurses learn about patients occurs because they are in an immediate and intimate relationship with the patient. This relationship exists because nurses provide intimate, bodily care. It is when a cancer patient is showering, and thus revealing her emaciated body, that she might confess,

"I am so thin, it is a wonder my husband can bear to look at me"—creating an opportunity to talk about her marital relationship and to consider ways of staying close when normal intimacy is impaired by illness.

It is when a nurse is drying her back that she will discover that a patient complains of pain over a thoracic vertebra, indicating early signs of spinal involvement and the potential for cord compression. This early recognition means the difference between being able to walk or being paralyzed. It is during a discussion of the symptoms arising from a new metastasis that the patient might talk about her increasing fears of approaching death: "I can't sleep at night as I fear I am going to die in my sleep." The nurse can then explore these fears and discuss with the patient and her family how important it is that she not be alone at night. In other words, the relationships that nurses form with their patients stem from their provision of basic physical care.

Basic nursing care is a euphemism for what the public often considers to be the distasteful—smelly, dirty, and unpleasant—aspects of nursing. It is frequently seen as unskilled work and is rarely valued in our society—either by the public or sometimes even by nurses themselves. Even patients who received skilled basic nursing care have limited capacity to articulate the positive impact this skilled work has had on them. Is it little wonder that some nurses tend not to value basic nursing care and are willing to hand it over to others?

Basic physical care allows issues to emerge that might not surface if nursing is limited to a formal set of questions delivered during a nursing assessment interview. The very intimacy of providing physical care to sick human beings allows the nurse to elicit details and engage in conversations that would otherwise be awkward to initiate. Nurses' ability to make critical assessments of patients' needs are so intimately bound up in basic care that nurses are unaware of making them and thus do not fully understand what is lost when physical care is handed over to others.

Occasionally, a story that describes how patients view the care they receive captures the importance of, and the skill involved in, basic nursing care. Dan Shapiro's book *Mom's Marijuana* includes an amusing but intensely moving account of his hospitalization following a bone marrow transplant. Early in his recovery, for the first time, he is feeling well enough to write. Full of hope, he is all set to begin when he drops his pencil. While bending to pick it up, he spills his urinal into his bed: "I felt as if a heavy, suffocating curtain had been dropped on me. In a heartbeat I went from feeling empowered and optimistic to thoroughly dehumanized . . . I felt frozen, weary, beaten down."[18]

He describes the arrival of a nurse who, with cool efficiency, changed his bed and gave him a fresh pencil, all with little fuss and certainly without causing embarrassment: "In the flap of a wing I was brought back. Restored."[19] This change of linen and pajamas may seem a routine and unimportant task, one that could have been delegated to an unskilled worker, but for Shapiro it had a much greater impact:

> With her practiced, gentle style, movements she made hundreds of times a day, she rehumanized me. I'm certain the number of times in my life I'll move, so quickly, between such radical extremes will be counted on one hand. But when I went back to thank her weeks later, she had no memory of the event. She politely acknowledged my thanks and smiled, awkward, looking away, not understanding the passion behind my praise.[20]

Shapiro is able to give voice to his experience in ways that illuminate the importance of what skilled nurses do at the bedside. His nurse undoubtedly would have understood that spilling a urinal is an embarrassing, even mortifying, experience and would have sought not to draw attention to it. However, such work is so routine that her ability to remember the specific instance may be limited. More critical, though, is whether she, or other nurses, understand how devastating such experiences can be and how much skilled care makes a difference to the patient. Most patients would have recounted this experience as an illustration of the nurse being kind and caring. Most would be unable to mobilize Shapiro's eloquence, or they might mention it and cover it with clichés—"the nurse is such a saint, an angel. I could never do that." Thus, the importance of such skilled care would be at best sentimentalized and at worst cloaked in silence and rendered invisible. If caring is central to nursing work, then we want nurses to have a positive effect on patients such as Dan Shapiro. If this is to happen, we must seek to understand and articulate this aspect and outcome of care. We must consider what is lost if we are unable to demonstrate how such care makes a difference to patients.

This clear articulation of basic nursing care is often difficult because nurses themselves do not find it pleasant or exciting to engage in basic nursing care when this requires working with excreta or bodily fluids. It is often hard work, and nurses are good at hiding the impact of what they do, both to protect the patient and others in their work environment. Nurses also believe that no one wants to hear the details about this kind of care. They are not taught how to describe these details in a way that enables those who are not nurses to appreciate the value of what are viewed as "disgusting jobs." Because it is so little rewarded and discussed, the major reward for the nurse is in knowing the patient felt clean and comfortable.

The following examples from a small study of nurses' experiences with malignant wound care illustrate the skilled work of nurses and how it is often discounted.[21] The patient, Mrs. J., had a cancer of the vulva that had fungated and spread to cover most of her abdomen. Taking off the dressing was very distressing for both the patient and the nurse. Nurse Jane Lawson described her ability to mask her own response to such a distressing wound and how important this masking was for the patient's well-being:

> LAWSON: "You guard your own reactions too. I mean with June I did guard my reactions and I watched my body language and everything very well, because the first thing was—my God, I don't believe I'm seeing this.
>
> RESEARCHER: "But you didn't say that?"
>
> LAWSON: "I don't want to, but how can I not—I don't want to put—it's not revulsion—but project my shock to her."
>
> RESEARCHER: "Why is it not revulsion? Why shouldn't it be revulsion?"
>
> LAWSON: "It's revulsion I suppose for the wound but not for the person, and you're dealing with the person, not just the wound."
>
> RESEARCHER: "So you are aware of your own body language and your own facial expression. You are doing that to protect the person?"
>
> LAWSON: "Yes. They have to live with it every day and it must affect their body image. And in fact it does. So you protect them and their sense of self that they are still a worthwhile person, even though they have this terrible wound.

We have no doubt that Mrs. J. would be able to describe the nurse's caring for her as kind and possibly even gentle. But would she be able to articulate the nurse's awareness of her distress? Would she understand how hard the nurse worked to normalize her experience by masking her own feelings of revulsion when taking off the wound dressing?

Another nurse, Tessa Fox, was caring for Mrs. A., who had a malignant wound on her sacrum that required daily dressings. She understood how unpleasant dressing changes were for Mrs. A., as well as for the nurses and the team. The wound was large and constantly drained an offensive-smelling discharge. As Nurse Fox described it:

> I can't begin to describe what was going on with this woman, but we got to the point where we were taking it in turns to go and see her each day and where possible doubling [sending two nurses] because it was just so hard. Someone could deal with this sobbing woman while the other person has got their head in this cavity in her backside trying to deal with the dressings and the bones and the filling it up and all the horrible things and so you didn't have to do two things at once.

Nurse Fox was able to capture several things in this story. She pointed to the way routine nursing care deals with the loss that accompanies bodily breakdown. She explained how she was able to deal with the distressed patient as she was simultaneously dressing the wound. She also talked about what she did when the wound became so large that normal procedures could no longer be used.

What is most interesting about her discussion of the care she gave patients with such wounds, and other examples of bodily breakdown, was how the multidisciplinary team dealt with her efforts to discuss this care in their regular meetings. When Nurse Fox began to talk about a patient's wound and the routine nursing care involved in changing dressings such as Mrs. A.'s, she found that the team tended to minimize it or to avoid it altogether. Team members asked Nurse Fox to "not give the gory bits" and began to groan when discussions of her work with patients contained too much detail. The team members that were not nurses dismissed it simply as that stuff nurses do, not very sophisticated and a bit yucky. Nurse Fox explained that the team rarely acknowledged this complex work:

> In the multidisciplinary team we start getting on to the wound stuff and we will say, sorry, we will talk about that later. Although I have deliberately sat down and told the whole team what we had to go through with Mrs. A. And I graphically described it and I have them nearly vomiting in their seats about what we had to go through every day, that assault on all five senses for two hours.

Unfortunately, Nurse Fox's response may not have increased the team's understanding of the skill involved in working with such bodily decay. As nurses seek to define their roles and responsibilities there is significant danger that aspects of care are seen as separate. Today many will argue that a technical specialist can do the dressing, a nurse's aide can shower the patient, and the palliative care case manager can help the patient adjust to their impending death and mobilize other aspects of the care team when other problems arise. We contend that it is in the nurse's ability to bring all of these aspects of care together (physical, technical, and psychosocial) and to understand and explain how they interact that nursing knowledge and skill becomes most visible.

The Complex Interplay between Physical, Technical, and Interpersonal Caring

The emphasis on psychosocial caring and the resultant changes in how nurses and their role are characterized is part of the overall development of nursing. However, acceptance of these changes without an ongoing critique can have unintended consequences—both positive and negative. Getting the balance right between the physical (doing), the technical (medical), and the psychosocial (talking) aspects of nursing, and understanding how they are linked, is crucial if nursing is to be a positive force in health care. Two stories from Sanchia Aranda's study of nurse-patient relationships help illustrate the various ways this interaction occurs in practice.[22]

This study of nurse-patient relationships drew on Annette Street's ideas about nurturance/knowledge.[23] It documented how, within close nurse-patient relationships, each nurse exercised power in ways that were responsive to the specific patient situation and aimed at making a difference. Street's work sought to move beyond negative portrayals of nurses exerting power over patients during care delivery—for example, by making the patient shower by 9 a.m. or by making intrusive demands for the disclosure of private matters—to make visible the ways in which nurses sought to use their knowledge of the patient to nurture them. In Aranda's study, the ability to make a difference arose from the interpersonal relationship that developed between the nurse and patient over various periods of time. In all situations the nurses said making a difference for patients was the tangible reward for doing a good job. The nurses placed little importance on public or professional recognition for their work, although when this occurred it reinforced the value of what they do. In almost all stories recounted for the study it was impossible to separate the physical, technical, and interpersonal dimensions of the effect nurses had on the patient's outcomes.

For example, Nurse Jasmine Barker, a nurse in a hematology unit, facilitated Mr. P.'s discharge from the hospital less than twenty-four hours before he died. Mr. P. had received a bone marrow transplant for a hematological malignancy. He now had liver complications that may have indicated advancing disease, an infection, or a complication of the transplant. The problem could not be precisely diagnosed without invasive tests, which Mr. P. was not well enough to undertake. The only condition amenable to treatment was the infection. Mr. P. was thus receiving antibacterial therapy that required hospitalization. Through discussions over many weeks, Nurse Barker delivered physical care and developed a relationship with Mr. P. He often confided how he was feeling. As Nurse Barker described it:

> The relationship with Mr. P. or someone else develops over such a long period of time, you are so in tune with every little difference in the person. You can sense changes in affect, physical changes, all sorts of things before anybody else does because you are there caring for them every day so inti-

mately. You know I could always sense a little bit of something different. Someone may hand over to me from the morning shift and I would be on the afternoon and "oh yeah, Mr. P.'s dah, dah, dah today" and I'd go in and I would see something completely different. Because I knew how he thought, how he felt about things, the way that he approached things day to day and pick up on those little changes, and that day I could just sense an urgency in him, that he needed to go home.[24]

As the antibacterial treatment continued Mr. P. told Nurse Barker that he was concerned the treatment wasn't working and that he wanted to die at home. Nurse Barker's knowledge of hematological malignancy and bone marrow transplantation led her to understand that Mr. P.'s concerns about the treatment were well founded. The treatment he was receiving for liver complications was potentially lifesaving if the symptoms were due to infection. However, if the complications were due to the cancer or to complications of the transplant then his current treatment would not be successful. Again, the cause of his current illness could not be identified with precision. Nurse Barker's ability to articulate to the medical staff the dissonance between the medical treatment plans and his desire to die at home was critical. It helped the medical staff alter his treatment and allowed him to receive treatment at home. Nurse Barker's actions were possible because of a complex interaction. She was able to forge a relationship with Mr. P. and gain knowledge of his wishes because of her knowledge of hematological malignancy and medical treatments. She had spent many days delivering intimate personal care including bathing and changing beds. She also performed a number of the technical practices (managing his chemotherapy and intravenous access). During all of this she was involved in a social interaction that allowed him to share his fears, life ambitions, and illness experience.

Nurse Barker's intimate knowledge of Mr. P. and her knowledge of hematological malignancy combined to create the nurturing she delivered to the patient. This also gave her the ability to balance treatment decisions with an understanding of Mr. P. the person as she discussed his care with the medical staff.

This story also emphasizes the relational basis of Nurse Barker's care of Mr. P. This relationship was constructed over time out of many different components and allowed her to shift gears when care of his psyche became more important than management of his disease. Medical management of complex disease situations is often a balance between costs and benefits, and the point at which the costs of treatment outweigh the benefits differs from person to person and is not always obvious. Nurse Barker's relationship with Mr. P. gave her insight into how he interpreted his situation through the many ups and downs during transplantation. Their relationship gave him a safe space to talk about his view of his situation, and from there Nurse Barker was able to convey his wishes to the medical team.

Hematological malignancy exemplifies how nursing management of the consequences of toxic treatments makes curative treatments possible. In treatment of hematological malignancy the aim is to kill cancer cells. The treatment, however, destroys the person's ability to make blood cells for a period of ten to fourteen days. During this time the patient is at risk of life-threatening infections and hemorrhage. The nurse's role is to closely observe early warning signs of infection or bleeding and to ensure the early initiation of appropriate therapy. Because it is usually the doctor's responsibility to order this therapy, the nurse is seemingly engaging in medical surveillance and reporting. In other words, she appears not to be a decision maker and critical thinker.

The reality is much more complex. The nurse is likely to have significant experience in monitoring patients for such treatment complications and will have an in-depth understanding of the medical actions required and the importance of early treatment. At least in a teaching hospital, the doctor is likely to be a junior member of the medical staff with little specialist knowledge in hematology. He or she will frequently depend on the nurse's experience in ensuring that appropriate treatment is initiated. Thus the nurse's caring work creates an important interface between the frequently changing junior medical staff and the medical management of patients with rapidly changing needs. In this case, the nurse is constantly making decisions and thinking critically.

The stories from this work on nurse-patient relationships also generated specific examples of how nurses mediate suffering through the provision of basic nursing care to people experiencing physical deterioration and decay. Human suffering was a key impetus for the development of the modern hospice movement. Hospice care has been portrayed as a reaction against inhumane treatment of people who were dying in a medical system that focused on the diseased body rather than the person.[25] The relief of suffering lies at the heart of palliative care, yet the literature on suffering in death and dying tends to give little prominence to the role of the body in suffering. The literature tends to focus on suffering as an existential experience with the bodily aspects of suffering inferred in descriptions of physical or emotional pain.[26] Although the link between suffering and the person's fear of being a burden is recognized there is little exploration of what "being a burden" means to patients.[27] Patients who dread becoming a burden fear they will no longer be able to clean themselves or carry out daily activities that keep them part of a family or social group. They fear not being able to hold their child or pick him or her up from school. They fear being smelly or incontinent. All of these signs of bodily breakdown contribute to, but are not fully understandable as, emotional distress. Similarly, the nursing work associated with helping the patient is easily discounted as only basic nursing care.

The story of Nurse Madonna Jenkins's care of Ms. Lucy Scully illustrates the ways in which the performance of seemingly basic nursing tasks, such as hygiene, offers an opportunity to nurture the spirit and psyche and ameliorate the suffering of those who are ill. Lucy Scully was a thirty-five-year-old model who was dying of a malignant brain tumor at home. Nurse Jenkins was the specialist palliative care nurse primarily responsible for her care, which occurred when direct patient care was a central part of the specialist palliative care nurse's role. Ms. Scully's illness resulted in significant physical changes, including lower limb paralysis and weight loss. The patient needed physical care such as assistance with bowel evacuation. Her physical deterioration had significantly affected her relationship with her husband, Paul, who felt unable to undertake her physical care. As Lucy became bed-bound and incontinent, Paul withdrew from physical contact with her and Lucy felt the loss of intimacy acutely. Nurse Jenkins describes her interactions with Lucy:

> I was really the only person who had the kind of relationship with her that I could spend time with her and actually listen to her fears and her feelings about what was happening. I don't think she did a lot of that with her husband, who found that very difficult, and her mother certainly wouldn't have, wasn't there, she couldn't be there at all emotionally or physically.
>
> That was really important to her because she could talk about all these issues with me, and then I did contribute in some way to her physical care. It was difficult, but in some way I tried to make it as dignified as possible against a whole lot of physical odds sometimes. I was able to recognize what was really important to her like getting up in the wheelchair and getting dressed in pretty clothes, putting on her makeup, that sort of thing. . . .
>
> There was a particular issue . . . just after she became bed-bound around intimacy with her husband. . . . After a few weeks of her being bed-bound and incontinent, he really withdrew from her and wouldn't touch her. Quite often he would sleep with her, but he was away from her. How painful that was for her, that she couldn't initiate anything with him, and how difficult it was for her that he didn't want to have sex with her anymore and that she had to have a catheter and that affected any of that anyway. . . .
>
> I did fulfil a little bit of that for her perhaps, some of that similar sort of intimacy stuff because I was touching her and massaging her and just generally being with her in a fairly sort of emotionally intimate space . . . how

important it was to put on makeup and still feel good about herself at the same time. . . . The extra time that I spent there was about helping her to do those things herself.[28]

In the intensely intimate times of providing basic nursing care for Lucy, Nurse Jenkins was able to meet some of her need for human touch. She was able to restore some of the patient's pride in her appearance, to discuss her feelings, and help ameliorate some of the distress inherent in such deterioration. Perhaps most important, she was able to offer the patient periods of normal human interaction with someone who was not disgusted by the changes she was enduring. How can the value of such interaction and care be assessed? Can it be easily dismissed as natural work requiring little formal education or knowledge? Would interpersonal interaction be as powerful if it were not combined with basic nursing care? In working with Lucy Scully, Nurse Jenkins drew on her knowledge of physiology (e.g., bowel care, prevention of pressure wounds), oncology (the spread of cancer and likely physical deterioration), psychology (e.g., understanding of personal experiences of approaching death, relationships), and sociology (the importance to humans of social interaction). The provision of basic nursing care was the ground on which this complex knowledge came together. Yet, when most nurses articulate their caring roles, do they do so in ways that illuminates the complexity of their care and knowledge? Is this how others understand what we do? Are most of us even aware of the impact of this work on those for whom we care? Do those who teach or manage nurses recognize this complex matrix and teach students how to describe it? Do those who construct nursing-image campaigns help nurses explain all of this to the public?

Rediscovering Bodywork: A Nursing Imperative

Our purpose in this chapter has been to show that caring in nursing is a complex interplay between knowledge drawn from a wide range of fields including medicine, psychology, and science. The setting in which nurses skillfully use this knowledge is the provision of basic nursing care to people unable to attend to many basic human functions independently during times of illness. Basic nursing care is critical to the ways in which nurses' work for several reasons. First, the very need for basic nursing care renders the patient vulnerable, which increases the extent to which the patient requires protection. The skilled nurse plays a critical role in ensuring the safety of patients unable to do this for themselves.

Second, the experience of vulnerability often leads patients to become willing to share the feelings and experiences that emerge when they are ill. A skilled nurse is able to gently explore this experience and to mediate the distress associated with being ill and vulnerable. Sometimes the nurse simply normalizes the patient's experience through her words and actions. At other times the nurse will draw on therapeutic communication skills to draw out the patient's fears and concerns, enabling a discussion of the strategies that can be used to address these concerns. This might be through the provision of health information or through evidence-based interventions known to successfully address such patient problems as pain, nausea, and fatigue.

Third, the skilled nurse's access to the patient's illness experience through basic nursing care enables her to influence patient outcomes. The nurse is able to understand the implications of seemingly unimportant details in the patient's experience and to use this information to influence medical treatment. This might include early identification of treatment complications such as infection or supporting the patient to discuss with their doctor the withdrawal of treatment that is becoming burdensome.

The stories recounted here provide rich illustrations of the complex work of nurses, which is often undertaken in private spaces with the patient, and highlight skills that are often hidden from view. The skill inherent in this work is not publicly understood, largely because the work itself violates social boundaries of what is acceptable to talk about. This work is also rendered invisible because the patient's vulnerability and the necessity to maintain patient confidentiality makes nurses feel they must remain silent in order to protect their patients. However, if nurses do not figure out a way to publicly express this private work without jeopardizing their patients, the profession itself will confront significant problems. One danger is that nurses themselves will continue to have limited ability to explain the importance of basic nursing care to themselves.

This is problematic for two reasons. Without an articulate understanding of the importance of basic nursing practice in the delivery of health care the skills used by nurses cannot be taught and valued in professional learning. This might deskill future generations of nurses who will be unable to integrate the complex knowledge that makes up nursing (particularly in the delivery of basic nursing care). This may result in negative consequences for patient outcomes.

More critically, nurses will not be able to influence those health policymakers who seek to cut costs by removing nurses from direct care and replacing them with seemingly less expensive and less-educated health workers. If nurses remain silent or do not adequately explain what the results of such policies might be, they will be complicit in policy changes that further remove them from basic nursing care. Nurses need to show that relationship and basic nursing care are not counterposed but intimately linked and that both the provision of emotional caring and basic physical care demand that nurses be not only clever but sometimes even brilliant.

If the threat to nursing is to be effectively confronted, nurses cannot disconnect themselves and their profession from the patients for whom they make a critical difference. "Clever nurses" are smart enough to care. If, as a profession, we pause and reflect on our history, we will remember and revalue the cleverness embedded in basic nursing. We also need to be cognizant of how this clinical intelligence rests on the critical interactions with patients that occur when nurses assist them with the basic necessities of life.

9

"You Don't Want to Stay Here"

Surgical Nursing and the Disappearance of Patient Recovery Time

Marie Heartfield

Mrs. Anu is an elderly woman who had surgery the previous evening for a fractured elbow sustained in a fall. As the nurse enters the room, Mrs. Anu, dressed with her bag packed, is trying to get back into bed. She picks up Mrs. Anu's notes from the end of the bed.

NURSE: Does your arm hurt? We can give you something for the pain. Yes, you are due, so I will get you something, okay?

MRS. ANU [*nodding as she reaches for the vomit bowl on the bedside table*]: Okay. I don't feel ready to go home. I am going to my daughter's but think I should stay; stay one more night.

NURSE: You'll be all right. You don't want to stay here, better to get home where your daughter can look after you; you'll feel better there.

MRS. ANU: You nurses say I have to go and I'll be all right. I suppose that I can ask my daughter to help me. I would just feel better having nurses and the doctor around. They know what is going on, my daughter doesn't. She is a nurse's aide in an old people's home, but she is off work with a bad back so I don't think I should go to her. There isn't anyone else. I am seventy-six years of age and live by myself. I would just feel better with the nurses and doctor around.

The story of Mrs. Anu comes from a study in which I observed nurses and patients frequently speaking at cross-purposes. Like many other patients in my study, Mrs. Anu attempted to negotiate a delay in her impending hospital discharge, because she did not feel ready to leave the security of the hospital following surgery. She felt frightened and unable to cope at home, and she worried about being a burden to her family. The nurse's response to these entreaties was to normalize, that is, to make the patient's problem and anxieties appear ordinary so there is no cause for concern. As she did so, she emphasized the value of home over hospital and thus implemented the institutional imperative to keep patient length of stay within set parameters.

The discussion between this nurse and patient, and my broader analysis of this phenomenon, emerges from a study of hospital length of stay in which I analyzed how changes in hospital length of stay shaped nursing and health care practices, as well as the way nurses think about patients, surgery, and recovery.[1] I studied hospital length of stay in the state of South Australia (1998–2001) by analyzing relevant national, state, and organizational policies and reports and through fieldwork that included observations and interviews with nurses, doctors, and patients in an acute surgical division of one urban hospital.

This analysis showed how ideas about surgical recovery were as much shaped by administrative discourses and concrete policies that had been reengineered to meet the hospital's need for short stays as they were by clinical discourses and practices that dealt with patient clinical status and progress. Discourse can be understood to be a "group of ideas or patterned ways of thinking which can be identified in textual and verbal communications while also located in wider social structures."[2] Critical understandings of discourses suggest that they work to undermine multiple meanings and produce, or emphasize, certain ideas, truths, or interests that derive from systems of knowledge and practices while shaping new ideas and practices. As lengths of hospital stay have become shorter, a literature of complaint, protest, and analysis has emerged. This literature critiques and analyses the phenomenon and assesses the consequences of shorter stays for patients.[3] The translation of length of stay to numbers of patients and to demand for hospital beds provides not only doctors and nurses but also patients, politicians, bureaucrats, and the media with a means to join the debate about what constitutes quality hospital services. This is evident in the widespread use of language about bed shortages and lengths of stay that is no longer restricted to health care professionals or hospital administrators.

As discussion of the global nursing crisis continues, the problem of shortened length of stay has become a topical one for nurses. There is a widely held view that decreased length of hospital stay decreases the quality of patient care. Some nursing literature suggests this happens through a diminished access to nursing, which changes the relationships between nurses and patients and makes it more difficult to provide appropriate care.[4] This discussion, however, usually casts nurses as unwilling victims of hospital budget cuts and the demands of hospital administrators. Nurses often argue that budget cuts force them to push patients through and out of the hospital "quicker and sicker." Nursing literature is thin on debates about the scientific, ethical, and economic aspects of managing clinical decision making; this is perhaps because clinical autonomy is usually attributed to the medical profession. Hence, there are few studies that examine these issues in relation to reductions in length of hospital stay and hospital throughput—that is, the focus on moving as many patients through the hospital admission period as possible.[5] Moreover, there is little discussion about how nurses themselves have embraced or facilitated hospital restructuring.

Many nurses have internalized the new policies of hospital and health care facility throughput. Even though hospitals provide professional nursing care, many nurses have become advocates of reduced hospital stays and thus reductions in the amount of professional nursing their patients receive. As one nurse in this study stated: "People just don't see the better service. We used to have a patient in bed for ten days; now we can have ten patients in a bed for one day each."

A failure to understand how nurses, like other health care workers, internalize the very values about which many of them complain obscures the power of dominant market modes of thinking. Nurses may actually be insulated against a more sophisticated understanding of this process as a result of internalizing the caring discourse that is so dominant in the field.

In the analysis I present here I do not intend a harsh or negative view of nursing practice. Rather, I question how nurses manage competing discourses, policies, and priorities. Nurses may believe that if they are caring, as many say they are, then they do not need a deeper involvement and participation in the market ideology and action associated with managing diminishing hospital lengths of stay. They may believe that because they continue to care and worry about the patients that they routinely and quickly process in to and out of the hospital, that this somehow moderates the implications of their daily actions.

Time as a Resource

The perceived changes in nurses' responsibilities toward the sick are a response to the fact that over the past decades in most industrialized countries hospital length of stay has been dramatically shortened. Patients who were in hospitals for ten days may now be in for three; patients who were in for three days may now be in only overnight; and many procedures that were once done in the hospital are being done in out-patient surgery centers where patients remain in the facility for only a few hours.

Suzanne Gordon calls the difficulty nurses have in providing high-quality health care—particularly face-to-face contact—a "mission impossible" for nursing.[6] Joan Liaschenko, writing in 1998 about changes in nursing knowledge, suggests that nursing has moved away from what nurses have often termed "nursing advocacy," defined as being able to speak on behalf of patients, to that of testimony, in which one now "bears witness to the event about which one speaks."[7] The contexts of decreased length of hospital stay and increased patient acuity mean that nursing may find itself with either far less or, at the very least, quite different things to testify about. Hospital nursing is being changed by the concept of time. In this sense, the nurse-patient relationship is being rewritten to remove the "relationship" aspect. It is now recast as an engagement "with service users within a tightly circumscribed time frame in order to accomplish the purpose at hand."[8] This is not to imply that nurses had previously, or traditionally, spent prolonged periods of time with individual patients or that some shifting of the burden of care to patients is not warranted. Nevertheless, the challenge is to understand how nursing practice is redefined in an environment in which changes in hospital reimbursement and policies are causing an overall diminished access to adequate nursing.[9] In response to the new challenge these changes create, a growing body of evidence documents that nurse-to-patient ratios and skill mix do make a significant difference to patients' hospital health care outcomes.[10] My aim in this chapter is to further explore this new dynamic and to help shape a response to it.

The Reconstitution of Hospitals

Acute care hospitals that emerged in the nineteenth century had as their goal providing a safe place for people receiving treatment as well as bed rest. For over a century, all across the globe, hospitals and hospital beds increased. Today, all over the world, the number of hospital beds per capita has decreased, although the rate of decline in hospital length of stay and hospital bed use is slowing.[11] The literature suggests that the deceleration in the decrease in hospital length of stay has occurred because cuts in length of stay have hit their peak and the increase in hospital admissions has been balanced by growth in the provision of out-patient treatments. Although there is an increase in the number of patients receiving out-patient care, the continued demand for hospital admission is attributable to the increasing numbers of older people and emergency admissions.[12] Hospital patients now go home from the hospital earlier, regardless of their reason for admission.

Analysis of what are relatively recent hospital innovations, including preadmission clinics and short-stay wards, suggests that the calculation of how much time a patient should spend in the hospital is losing significance as attention shifts to the patient's responsibility for his or her own care. Patients are now informed in preadmission clinics about what will happen during and after their hospital stay.

In a parallel development for nurses, not only the time the patient spends in the hospital but the hospital bed has become central to how they define their management mission. For nurses and administrators alike, hospital beds are familiar as fixed central places of hospital care. Nurses maintain them in detailed and specific ways as the visible, central, and observable places of patient care and nursing practice. Hospital beds are also considered in economic terms and are perceived to be expensive. In addition, when considered in terms of rates of hospital-acquired infection, hospital beds have become risky, or perhaps even dangerous, locations for care and treatment. The effect of developments such as bed-management programs and preadmission clinics in structuring the demand for hospital beds also assists in managing clinical uncertainty. Previously, hospital discharge was a result of clinical judgment rather than a compounding factor in patient throughput. This has changed because the work done in the preadmission and short-stay areas predetermines discharge timing, which lessens the need for nurses and doctors to consider this issue.

Further evidence of the reshaping of contemporary hospitals can be seen in specialized units and new areas of nursing expertise. These new units are often specifically designed to achieve shorter lengths of stay through separating patients by anticipated duration of stay rather than by biomedical specialty. These developments have an impact on areas of practice that nurses have begun to claim as specializations; for example, wound care, out-patient surgery, and convalescence. Just as the clinical specialties of medicine are now forced to compete with the managerialist reframing of hospital spaces, so these nursing specializations have also become fragile. In environments of decreasing patient stay, nurses become specialists not only in clinical areas of biomedicine but in organizing patient throughput, such roles as "bed manager," "discharge liaison," or "home care nurse."

With hospitals increasingly redefined as being appropriate only for people requiring acute biophysical intervention, chronic illnesses and social needs that were formerly met by hospitalization have become problems for communities to handle. They often pose problems for nurses, whose work had previously focused on this complex mix of needs.

Recasting of the Surgical Event

Patients that undergo acute surgical care will experience many "recoveries." Nurses care for these patients from the time they regain consciousness after general anesthesia to their return to pre-illness states. Nurses in this study considered their role to be "the minimization of trauma." Thus, they worked with patients to identify real or potential problems, needs, and risks, and to find ways to address them. A successful way to achieve this for elective surgical patients was to have them attend a hospital clinic before surgery (preadmission clinic) where they would meet separately with nurses, surgeons, and anesthetists. Through these consultations, the surgical event was "normalized" and regulated by getting patients to identify and understand how they could manage more of their own health care. Access to hospital beds was also managed, as nurses worked with patients to keep hospital stays brief. Length of stay thus became a social and political mode of control or "government." The word "government" in this context relates to Michel Foucault's concept of governmentality and the shaping of human conduct and management of populations through power operating in various ways at various sites.[13]

In the preadmission and short-stay areas, nurses worked with patients to teach them about what would happen before and after surgery. They counted on these sessions to help patients understand that they had a responsibility to care for themselves. Patients were helped to identify any existing self-care needs and were encouraged to be ready to manage the needs that would occur after surgery. Nurses, and to a lesser degree doctors, made it clear that a patient's needs had to adapt to and fit in with what could be provided by the hospital. Thus, self-care supplemented hospital health care services.

We see this in the case described at the beginning of this chapter. Mrs. Anu confronted her nurse with a number of options and interpretations that the nurse seemed unwilling to consider. She describes herself as being unable to leave the hospital, because she is not well enough (she feels sick and faint); not organized enough (her plans for leaving are not yet finalized); and does not have access to adequate care, expertise, and resources. She does not want to go to her daughter's: her daughter has worked in an old persons' home, but she lacks the expertise of the nurses and doctor; she has a bad back, thus should not, or cannot, be expected to care for her mother; and Mrs. Anu doesn't know when her son-in-law can get to the hospital to take her home. The nurse reinterprets, or ignores, these comments as she searches through alternative reasons to explain why Mrs. Anu needs to accept her impending hospital discharge. "Rest" and "something for the pain" are suggested, but only after these symptoms are situated within a time frame of "going home this morning." Sharing in the aim of "getting the patient going," Mrs. Anu had packed her bags and has tentatively arranged her transport home. The nurse at handover to other nurses describes this patient as having a "history with anesthetics," which suggests that it is normal, as in okay, for her not to tolerate anesthetics well. Nausea and dizziness are common, therefore predictable, responses to anesthetic drugs. Even though the nurse is familiar with this kind of response and Mrs. Anu had experienced these symptoms with a prior hospitalization, it was unlikely that Mrs. Anu's experience had made her current one less difficult for her. When the nurse normalized her symptoms in this way, she indicated that Mrs. Anu's problems were not significant and that they could be easily managed through rest and analgesia. Indeed, she suggested that they would be even less of a problem at home.

Even though some analgesics commonly exacerbate postanesthetic symptoms of nausea and dizziness, the nurse insists that home is a better place for Mrs. Anu than the hospital. She told Mrs. Anu that her symptoms did not justify (or permit) a continuation of her hospital stay. Mrs. Anu countered with reasons it was inappropriate for her to stay with her daughter. For the nurse, however, not to be in the hospital—no matter how problematic the site—was to be "at home." Nursing practice in this instance was adhering to an administrative imperative from the hospital that patient episodes of care take place within the predicted length of stay. The nurse succeeded in following the hospital protocol and discharging the patient within the set time frame by "normalizing" the patient's symptoms.

The dialogue between Mrs. Anu and the nurse makes visible another dimension. Attention to hospital length of stay not only influences nurses and others to pay attention to how long patients stay in hospital but it also shapes nurses' belief that patients are well enough before surgery to allow hospital discharge to be predicted in advance of the surgical procedure. This, even though these patients have conditions that require surgery and often have preexisting conditions that can complicate recovery. Nevertheless, the processes of hospital admission and hospital discharge are now fused in time.

Previously, when doctors and nurses made decisions about a patient's recovery and care needs, they did so after making clinical assessments and judgments while the patient was recovering from the procedure. Today, before the patient even has his or her surgery, the after-care period is determined. A new kind of patient has emerged in the discourse and in practice—a patient who is understood to be "prerecovered." This prerecovered patient eliminates, except in extreme cases, the requirement that doctors and nurses make clinical assessments during the postoperative period, as the plan for the patient has already been developed. Only serious complications warrant a break in the preset schedule. It is up to the nurse, not the patient, to determine what constitutes a serious complication.

Rationalities and Consequences

In the new market model, recovery is understood in terms of length of hospital stay, and the patient's understanding of his or her resources for self-care has been completely redefined. Surgical recovery is not limited to a continuous postoperative time or space; instead, it moves between the before and after, the public and the private, the hospital and the home, and the available and accessible. In this space, patients are "recast as rational, responsible, knowledgeable and calculative."[14]

Allocation of a hospital bed, and movement in to and out of that bed, are recognized as indicators of a patient's health status.[15] The process of making decisions about hospital admission and allocation of people to hospital beds appears to be a straightforward one. At the same time, hospital admission involves the complex organization of paradoxical patient-care issues. Patients are required to cooperate with the demands of the health care system and accept that they need to be able to know about, and provide for, their own recovery.

The calculation of length of stay is not only evident in architectural changes to hospitals such as the addition of short-stay and preadmission areas. It is also found in the information gathering and calculation that is integral to hospital reengineering of bed management, early discharge, and home care. Length of hospital stay also features in less obvious discursive and practical activities through which economic and therapeutic efficiencies combine to strengthen the social requirement for self-care. Along with beds, the patient experience of recovery has become the territory of health care policies and practices. The "success" of these policies and practices is now understood as being governed through the production of new truths, truths that moralize individual recovery.

Preadmission and the Perfect Hospital

The social constructions and policies that determine care in preadmission and short-stay areas illuminates the new thinking about patients. Following surgical diagnosis, the care that patients are allocated is linked to their predicted length of stay rather than to assessment of their clinical response or need. One nurse (Nurse Karen) said, "I think the preadmission clinic is one of the best things. If every patient could come through there, probably the hospital would be perfect." For this nurse, the perfect hospital is produced in the preadmission process, which furnishes nurses with ways of understanding that create particular ideas about patients. As an entry point to the hospital, the preadmission clinic in turn directs how nurses practice.

The nurses doing patient assessments and interviews in the preadmission clinic also worked on the various surgical wards. These same nurses would help care for these patients after their admission to the hospital and after their surgeries. The preadmission unit process was viewed as useful because, as the same nurse said, "We get to see them while they are still well. I mean I know they need surgery, but in the preadmission unit they are usually fit and well and this helps to know what they should be like after they have had their surgery." Just as surgeons and anesthetists share a biomedical discourse that requires patients to both need surgery and "be fit" for anesthesia,[16] so do patients seeking admission to the hospital need to be "fit" and "well" although in need of surgery. Nurses in this analysis were involved in thinking about, engaging with, and securing care for, individual patients. Simultaneously, they had to comply with organizational structures and processes consistent with "a perfect hospital," which is now understood as a hospital with a predicable patient length of stay.

In the preadmission clinic, nurses conducted assessments and interviews with the patient and, when they were present, with family and friends. In various ways, nurses told patients that "to be ready for discharge we need the wound to look good, no temperature, have you eating and drinking, and for you to be up and able to move around" (Nurse James).

Although nurses often mentioned that the conditions for hospital discharge appeared to depend on assessment of clinical or functional conditions, an anticipated length of stay was always included in their considerations. In the preadmission interview nurses commonly talked to patients about their anticipated length of hospital stay. As the following examples illustrate, this communication was usually of quite a directive nature: "This type of surgery needs two or three days" (Nurse James). "This type of surgery only needs one or two nights" (Nurse Gail). The nurses' reference to length of stay in their preadmission consultations subtly signaled to patients and to those accompanying them that the length of their hospital stay was as significant as their clinical condition. As Nurse Pauline put it, "Short stay, long stay, they are really quite different things. The whole process for these patients depends on how long we think, or I should say know, really, as these days we pretty well know exactly how long they will be here." Despite their desire to create the perfect hospital, nurses commonly spoke to patients in ways that affirmed that the hospital was an unfavorable place to be: "The whole idea of this [preadmission] clinic is to get all of the preoperative care done before you're admitted. All the things we used to do after you came in to hospital we now do beforehand so you don't have to be here for as long. It's better as you get home quicker" (Nurse Gail).

Nursing Strategies for Managing Hospital Length of Stay

One of the key strategies in the preadmission unit involved the exchange of information. This involved the scrutiny of the patient's body for confirmation of disease or of the symptoms necessitating surgery and of fitness for anesthesia. It also focused on providing patients with information about their surgery and what they needed to do to prepare for it. Nurses took notes on the patient's expectations of the scheduled surgery, social and home circumstances, and daily or regular activities such as lifestyle and occupation. Gathering information about the patient's personal and social circumstances made what was previously invisible to nurses, and often to patients, visible, such as patient anxiety, pain management experiences, and home help. These were all factors that might negatively affect the length of the hospital stay:

> The preadmission patients are different; well, for one, they know all about the operation, the doctors have gone down there, the nurse goes too, but often it's the actual consultant [senior hospital doctor] that goes down and speaks with the patient. They [the patients] understand the operation, they understand all the postoperative expectations of the nursing staff and medical staff and things like that; they know what has to be done, and we know all about them. We know their social situation and their home situation so there are no issues about them not being able to go home on time. (Nurse Carol)

This constitution of the "preadmission patient" aligns with a rationality of the perfect hospital through processes of "they know" and "we know." The patient and the nurse were made visible through information strategies that highlighted what the patient knows and what the nurse knows. On the one hand, the patients know all the postoperative expectations; that is, the patients know what is required of them in the impending hospital surgical episode. On the other hand, the nurses know all about them; that is, the nurses have been able to learn, and document for others, the necessary details to predict discharge and the movement of the patient through the surgical episode. In the following discussion we will see how these techniques produce various roles and identities for nurses and patients.

Resourcing and the Resourced

Nurses limited the allocation of hospital resources through working on, and with, patients to identify self-care resources so that self-care resources can be substituted for what has been defined as scarce hospital resources. These practices helped solve real or potential problems by "identifying" the necessary resources.

Nurses have always needed comprehensive clinical knowledge about a wide range of surgical interventions as well as the process of recovery. Nursing competence now includes the prediction and control of length of patient stay. In this study, nurses described the skills that they had to master as being able to "get them [patients] through [the hospital]" or to "get them going." The identification of patient circumstances that might interrupt quick and predictable hospital throughput, and hence avoid "bed blockers," was important.[17] A valued nursing competence was the "practices of resourcing." Significantly, the success of this process required nurses and patients to have shared expectations of surgery and recovery.

A key aim for nurses in the preadmission consultations was establishing whether patients had social networks (family members or friends). As patients described people with whom they lived, or those they considered might help them after discharge from the hospital, nurses framed these individuals as "carers," even if they were ill equipped to provide caregiving. Examples of carers included not only the willing and able but also spouses with dementia, young children, and adults who were disabled. As is evident in the earlier scenario with Mrs. Anu, the resourcing of patients continued after surgery. In the process, patients' responses or concerns about discharge—such as pain, nausea, and vomiting—were discounted, or reframed as normal and, thus, self-manageable.

Preadmitted and Prerecovered

Recovery for individuals in this study involved thinking, description, calculation, and prediction about the details of the surgical event, and was considered in the context of the availability of public and private resources. This involved a shift in the diagnosis of recovery. Because the guiding premise was that the patient was *well*, there was less discussion, concern, and perhaps even acknowledgment of uncertainty about how individual patients progressed after surgery. The period of postoperative observation was reduced, and the work of managing recovery (through identifying resources) was done before the surgery. Recovery shifted from an emphasis on postoperative assessments and the treatment of somatic, or psychic, responses to a focus on whether patients or their families knew how to manage responses or where to get help elsewhere to manage problems.

Through assumptions about the patient's capacities for self-care, surgery was "normalized," that is, turned into something a nonprofessional could successfully navigate. However, this *self-care* was not necessarily health care as it may previously have been understood. Only certain types, or levels, of recovery could occur within the hospital setting. With the exception of some elderly individuals, few patients in this analysis could influence the duration of their hospital stay. Moreover, patients were rarely taught how to manage their lives in ways to avoid further sickness or ill health. Although nurses pride themselves on being patient educators, this role was narrowed to the point of invisibility. Nurses instructed patients only about things that pertained to recovery from the surgical episode. In environments where hospital patients are recognized as having multiple chronic illnesses, the planning and care associated with surgical episodes was often managed as though they were isolated and separate from existing health conditions.[18] Consequently, surgical care in this health service was separated out as an isolated intervention, which is clearly at odds with the holistic approach to health care.[19] Though some nurses expressed frustration at their inability to practice in the more comprehensive manner they thought appropriate and necessary, other nurses spoke confidently of this narrowing of attention as indicative of an emerging era of specialization.

Determining whether a patient was fit and well did not take place following surgery, nor did it occur as part of the daily examination of the patient's condition. In fact, the definition of the patient as well and therefore able to assume self-responsibility for their health care on discharge occurred *in advance* of both surgery and recovery. In asking patients to take responsibility for their own health, nurses expected patients to be able to function as rational actors who would, of course, act according to the rewritten health care script of short hospital stays.[20] At the same time, however, patients' behavior was tightly regulated in ways that served the needs of the hospital and state. The primary goal was to produce patients who were what Gordon calls "predictable units of production."[21] Furthermore, these patients moved in and out of the hospital in a predetermined fashion, so that hospital beds could be efficiently managed, which rendered redundant nursing ideals about time-dependent, holistic, and therapeutic relationships between nurses and patients.

The shrinking duration of hospital stays requires health systems (and seemingly also nurses) to have particular ideas about socially accepted sick roles. For instance, hospital systems rely on patients to be independent and stay in the hospital only as long as it takes for them to learn the necessary "new ways" of caring for themselves. In this way hospital patients are categorized through information exchanges (they know/we know) that enact the expertise of the nurse (to resource them) and the patient (to resource themselves). This reorganization of the nursing role away from doing things for patients toward teaching them how to do things for themselves not only accommodates the needs of hospital rationalizers for shortened hospital stays but may also alleviate some of the problems that stem from the global shortage of hospital nurses.

Nursing Reconfigured

Aileen Clarke and Rebecca Rosen suggest that the reduction in hospital length of stay requires a shift in focus from the place of care—that is, the hospital or home—to the components of care.[22] Although there are many examples of the difficulties experienced by former patients and their carers after shortened hospital stays, systematic research reviews tell us that, with the exception of the very old and the very young, there are minimal biophysiological problems with shorter hospital stays.[23] The organizational consequences of the decreasing length of hospital stay are measured only through readmission to the hospital for reasons specifically related to the same episode of care, such as for a wound infection. Although it may appear that there is a presumption that individual experiences after discharge from the hospital are unimportant and inconsequential to health care efficiencies, the decreasing length of hospital stay underlines the problems with a focus on biophysiology and the need for greater attention to understanding the impact on overall patient outcomes. As this study showed, patients may not have suffered more complications or even been readmitted to the hospital, but they did exhibit significant concern about being discharged early from the hospital.

To date nursing research has not documented a connection between reduced length of stay and serious patient harm; it does confirm the validity of nurses' concerns about workload, understaffing, and overwork. Such research also suggests that it is becoming increasingly difficult for nurses to construct therapeutic relationship and to practice time-dependent, holistic care. Moreover, nurses' focus on these ideals often lacks grounding in a clear description of contemporary nursing and health care practice. More research is needed to communicate the difference that such ideals make to patient outcomes if policymakers, politicians, managers, and other members of the health care team are to understand why it is important to realize such ideals.

Current schemes to decrease the duration of hospital stay, especially for surgical patients, demand that nurses consider their role in the diagnosis and delivery of such "components of care."[24] Nursing practice is now understood as consisting of "time limited interventions."[25] Nurses who work in an era of shrinking length of hospital stay are busy managing the care requirements that come with increased hospital patient acuity. They are also involved in a closer scrutiny and diagnosis of the resources needed to implement a decreased length of stay. With the increasing brevity and potential risks of hospital stays, knowledge about what is involved in health care episodes and the human experiences of illness and recovery may well be at risk.

Organizational inefficiencies and the dynamics of medical authority previously resulted in hospital stays that were often longer than necessary, and lengths of stay are now radically shortened. Indeed, by sending home the patients who are deemed to have fewer needs for "low intensity nursing care days," self-help has become a substitute for professional nursing. What is interesting is how nurses have internalized this position.[26]

Policymakers and the system as a whole have succeeded in restricting bed occupancy time (hence patient visibility and need) by redefining surgical recovery as mundane and predictable. Nurses actively promote shifting the burden of care to patients and to their family carers, who bear the responsibility for care or self-care, as they attribute to patients hitherto unrecognized capacities for that kind of care. At the heart of this dynamic is a process through which nurses shift from doing things for patients to teaching patients how to do things for themselves. Despite recognition of the impact of this cost and activity shifting to carers and communities, we do not know enough about the consequences of this trend.[27] For example, how do current developments in surgical technique, and the associated changes to hospital surgical systems, shape health care knowledge (for both providers and consumers)? We know that increasingly sophisticated surgical technology has decreased the potential for complications and increased the demand for surgery. However, what does it mean when surgery is viewed as an isolated health event that is deemed to exist in a vacuum?

New Moralities of Nursing Practice

Florence Nightingale suggested that "a hospital should do the sick no harm."[28] Contemporary definitions of nursing still value the tasks "of looking after people when they are too ill to look after themselves, and to wean them back to self care as they recover."[29] If the ideal of "doing no harm" is to be relevant and enacted in everyday practice, it will only occur when hospitalized patients are recognized and conceptualized as being sick in the first place. It cannot happen if people sick enough to need surgical intervention are redefined as not being sick.

Today, however, patients are discouraged from becoming dependent on nursing care. If they do need care, they are quickly weaned off nursing care and oriented toward self-care. This occurs through resource creation, rather than resource referral. Nurses and patients discuss the patient's "postsurgical needs" and how they can be managed—a discussion that also considers who at home can help them manage. They were rarely told about health care resources in which services are delivered to them by qualified professionals in a hospital or institutional setting: they were told about resources they themselves could provide or that they could access in the community. When one delves more deeply, these interactions were somewhat contradictory. Patients were expected to be both responsible and self-caring, yet they were expected to unquestioningly accept the direction of health experts.

Sick, dependent patients are encouraged to accept this requirement for self-management and self-control. Through this process, their experience of surgery is brought into line with the priorities of policymakers and financial interests that are now limiting what governments provide for individuals. Hence, length of stay is part of a calculated approach to economic organization of hospital services. Such practices challenge the nursing profession to join the broader public debate about health services. We need to be cognizant of the ways in which this debate and the resultant policies have the capacity to reshape our practice and to influence our relationships with patients and their families and carers.

In these times of limited social health funding and shrinking hospital stays, nurses, as a professional group, run the considerable risk of becoming either overwhelmed by, or desensitized to, the broader implications. In their comments below, two nurses illustrate the difficulty in attempting to balance organizational demands with connecting with, and doing things for, the patients they care for:

> I am pretty busy this morning. I've got Mr. Jones. He needs full nursing home care. Later today he'll be transferred back [to the nursing home], but this morning I have to fully feed and shower him. We're just not set up for that here [in a short-stay ward]. Four of my beds already have their second patient for the day in, and by the time I go home some of them will have even a third. We just can't care for people like that. (Nurse Jane)

> We manage through teamwork, though I don't like it when a patient comes in and then goes off to [surgical] theater before I have had a chance to meet them. I am each patient's nurse. I am the one looking after them on that day, and if I am looking after them then I like to be able to do things, like to get them ready for theater. I get really concerned about the patients, because that is what we are here for. Even though things get done and organized, from a ward point of view it is not right, it is not what I call nursing if they don't even know who is looking after them, if I can't do some things for my patients. (Nurse Meri)

Disturbingly, such instrumental observations demonstrate nursing's increasingly limited insight into patients' needs, and arguably they highlight a wider social desensitization to sickness!

Previous hospital and patient-care studies have indicated problems with the disease, sickness, and institution-oriented focus of hospital care. The primary health care movement that emerged with the Declaration of Alma-Ata and the Ottawa Charter attempted to shift health services away from sickness and toward prevention and self-responsibility.[30] However, the move by many governments away from a focus on the individual and toward communities and other groups attests to the fact that maintaining health is often beyond the scope of the individual and requires the addition of global ideals and actions.[31] In my analysis I am not arguing against what might be seen as an appropriate de-emphasis on hospital care and a focus on home and community care. I do, however, question taken-for-granted contemporary notions that hospitals are risky and unpleasant places, and that patients are far better off at home. The idealization of "home is best" is based on assumptions about the availability of health workers with knowledge and skills, in addition to someone available to take care of the sick patient, not to mention the economic resources of food and shelter. This is not to diminish the incidence of hospital-acquired infection and the growing realization that hospitals are not necessarily safe or pleasant places to be; nor does it suggest that economic resources should be made available for health care systems to meet every patient's every need.

Length of Stay: A Disappearing Rather Than Diminishing Influence

In nursing practice and patient care, length of stay has become a rigid standard. It sets norms not only for data-reporting purposes but also establishes the norms governing the behavior of nurses and patients. In this way, length of stay is part of new governable spaces—spaces now subject to state intervention and control. These new spaces make possible the extension of authority as part of the discursive and practical classification and calculation of hospital (and bed) use. Although patients, nurses, doctors, consumer activists, and many others have attempted to reconcile their expertise with the various and competing clinical and managerial discourses and policies, length of stay has shifted from numerical outcome "facts" to a delineation of individual responsibilities. The ease with which health professionals translate the phrase "length of stay" into an obligation to notice how long a patient has been in the hospital or, better still, to seek to decrease that period of stay, is evidence of this.

Nurses that I interviewed suggested that in short-stay surgical areas they did not have enough time to care. Simultaneously, they argued that the hospital was not always the best place to be. Nurses sometimes reclassified surgical patients as "elderly" so that a patient might be able to stay in the hospital longer. In this process, the bed ceases to be a therapeutic space where medical or nursing care is practiced and becomes instead a mobile administrative space. Nurses' sphere of responsibility is increasingly focused on the duration of bed occupancy. Nursing practice in this analysis involved ensuring that patients could find the resources to do for themselves without the hospital. This is an activity and preoccupation that coincides not only with managerialist agendas but also with contemporary agendas of risk management and social responsibility.

The Lightning of Possible Storms

Length of stay is clearly more than a neutral, calculated, and numerical hospital outcome. It is one of the strategies through which the work of decreasing hospital length of stay and increasing the volume of patients—that is hospital throughput—is accomplished. As it attracts attention and directs resource use in preadmission and short-stay programs, length of stay has ceased to be a means to an end and has become an end in itself.

The focus on length of stay is part of a process that produces new knowledge about beds and responsibilities for self-care. This new knowledge has the potential to erode what surgical nurses have previously known about what it means to be sick. To use this new knowledge about beds and re-sponsibilities—particularly in an era when they are overwhelmed with in-creased patient load and acuity—some nurses need to forget what it is they know and consider why they have been asked to provide care to those who are unwell. These developments require further examination.

Nursing has always been a dynamic and evolving profession. It has al-ways responded to new developments in health care delivery and to shifts in the global workforce. Today, however, the main issue is not whether nursing is changing. The question to be asked is changing into what?

10

Research on Nurse Staffing and Its Outcomes
The Challenges and Risks of Grasping at Shadows

Sean Clarke

When contemporary nurses talk about their ability to care for patients, a recurrent theme emerges: they are so short staffed on hospital floors, many say, that they don't have time to give basic physical care and have even less time to give the emotional care most nurses consider the hallmark of quality nursing. Some feel that the ability of nurses to plead the case for improved staffing relies on nurse researchers demonstrating that good staffing levels have a positive effect on patient care. The body of research literature dealing with the effects of nurse staffing has grown rapidly since the mid-1990s, when there was virtually no published research documenting a connection between staffing levels and patient outcomes.[1] As of this writing in 2005, there are several dozen studies that point to a connection between staffing and safety in hospitals. The picture emerging from this research is clear: poor patient outcomes tend to be more common in hospitals and on nursing units where staffing levels are low, that is, where nursing staff are responsible for more patients on average.[2]

These studies have had a major impact on the nursing profession and have influenced public perceptions of nursing work around the world, no doubt because they follow and amplify worrying reports of a large and deepening shortage of nurses in many Western countries. Their message hits a special chord with a public already witnessing changes in hospitals and told to expect worsening staffing. They also resonate with nurses as well as hospital officials and government leaders responsible for ensuring

Preparation of this chapter was assisted in part by K01-NR07895, National Institute of Nursing Research, United States National Institutes of Health.

patient safety in a climate of financial constraints. Overall, the papers are read as both a validation of nursing's role in hospital safety and as a call for hospital officials and politicians to act.

However, the influence of the staffing literature is not as widespread as it could be because of disconnects between care in daily practice, on one hand, and what researchers are able to measure, on the other. Readers of this literature must make many intuitive leaps to apply these studies to the real world, because the average patient and the average nurse in these studies are constructions of researchers and don't exist in clinical practice. Furthermore, researchers are able to say very little about the direct effects of staffing on safety, since the evidence that connects staffing with outcomes is largely circumstantial.

It is time for staffing research to more directly address the substance of nursing—skilled and competent care provided within the nurse-patient relationship. Staffing researchers have extensively studied the shadows of nursing or the traces of nurses' work left behind in the operations of health systems. Such shadows are found in payroll records and institutional budgets and in incidence rates for commonly recorded outcomes that raise questions about possible lapses in care. Although these data, however imperfect, have been key to enormous progress in the field, they do not capture the essence of what nurses do for their patients. Furthermore, there are many dangers in crudely quantifying nursing services.

Research findings on staffing and safety have attracted attention and opened dialogue in ways few thought possible even five years ago. However, they fall short in addressing pressing practical questions about managing nurse human resources. Endless grasping at nursing's shadows could have dire consequences for the profession. Relying on current data sources is a risky strategy for demonstrating that safe care is based on judgment as well as physical labor and task completion. Findings generated with data stripped of their practice context could undermine nurses' long fight to help the public recognize that their profession must be practiced under conditions that support knowledge work. Losing the substance of nursing might also have very unfortunate consequences for the public if it leads to short-sighted managerial and policy decisions at a time of unprecedented turbulence in the nurse labor market. If manipulating the quantity of nurses working in health care systems continues to be the target of policy and regulatory decisions without considering the factors influencing nurses' functions in the delivery of care, many countries could end up within several decades with nurse workforces that do not meet their societies' needs.

Nursing outcomes research is targeted at two audiences. The first is inside the profession. This group seeks to understand why patients do well or poorly under different circumstances and wants to improve systems of care. The second is an audience outside the profession that uses outcomes research data to direct health policy, particularly in funding services and programs. Staffing research has overcome major methodological challenges and has had a considerable influence in both groups. The research has been widely read and has changed the nature of discussions about patient safety and nurse workforce issues. However, taking the next steps that will inform resource allocation decisions inside and outside the profession will require innovative thinking. It will require returning the essence of nursing practice to its rightful place at the center of discussions about the responsible management of nursing resources, as well as careful thinking about the uses and limits of research data in decision making. It will also necessitate some soul-searching regarding the values questions underlying personnel allocation decisions.

Staffing research and the nursing profession are at a crossroads. If researchers continue to grasp at the shadow of nursing work instead of at the essence of nursing practice, diminishing returns on scientific efforts can be expected. In the worst-case scenario, the profession's efforts to provide high-quality services may ultimately be sabotaged. In this chapter I review some of the challenges and dilemmas facing researchers and the profession and address two broad questions: How and in what ways is it challenging to link staffing research with clinical reality? What are the causes and consequences of disconnects between research and practice? The "question behind the question" is a simple one, where next? In what directions should staffing research now proceed? How should leaders and policymakers apply this body of research? The points raised are intended to provoke reflection and discussion among readers of this literature, researchers seeking to design the next generation of studies on staffing and outcomes, and all those attempting to map the future of the profession.

How Well Does Staffing Research Reflect Clinical Reality?

Researchers face recurring problems in measuring the concepts that interest them. Three questions face researchers every time they design studies: Is it theoretically possible to measure concepts of interest? Are there accepted techniques for measuring them? Can any available measures be applied across enough different patients or patient-care settings to enable research studies to be carried out? The gaps between what researchers wish to understand ("patient safety," "quality of care," and "adequate staffing" are three good examples) and what they are able to measure can be enormous. However, even when measurement tools tested in previous research can be located, the costs of obtaining data on the measures (whether surveying patients, observing care, or drawing data from existing sources) can force compromises in the scope of studies.

As a result, researchers can sometimes use data sources and measurement techniques to directly measure what interests them, but often the variables available for use are some distance away from the heart of the matters involved. Suppose a group of researchers wants to know whether the nursing time particular patients are receiving matches the patients' needs for care. The research team will often settle for examining easily obtained statistics that divide the number of work hours for registered nurses in a hospital by the number of patients cared for (in the form of patient-days) over a year. They do this because no other data are available on a sufficiently large scale that would reveal whether the treatment needs of patients were satisfied. The result is a clear divide between the intent and the measures selected. The gap between the concepts of real interest and the variables available for analysis is called "conceptual slippage." Staffing research is not alone in facing conceptual slippage and other measurement problems; an ironclad requirement in applied research for one-to-one correspondence between the variables and the concepts of interest would quickly bring research to a halt. Still, it is essential to keep slippage in mind and to exercise caution when interpreting research results. Sometimes, because advocates of various positions in nursing are deeply committed to certain stances, they overlook slippage and related problems in the research they believe supports their points of view.

A deeper understanding of what staffing research has established (and what it has yet to establish) begins by examining the elements common to all studies in this field. Let's take a closer look at the two major variables, staffing and patient outcomes, as well as what is known about the mechanisms that tie the two together.

Measuring Staffing

Staffing levels are an expression of the numbers of nursing staff providing care to specific groups of patients over particular time periods. They are ratios of some unit of nursing work (hours of professional nurses' time, for instance) to some unit of service (a patient-day, for example).

Staffing can be measured across an entire institution or a specific nursing unit. Staffing statistics may or may not take into consideration workers other than fully qualified professional nurses and they may or may not incorporate nursing personnel who do not deliver care at the bedside.[3] Generally speaking, currently used staffing measures obliterate differences across the nurses and the units and shifts where they are assigned. In most, if not all, studies, patient-days too are analyzed as equivalent to each other. There are enormous differences between caring for patients who present for care under straightforward conditions and experience normal courses of disease and recovery, and caring for patients who are complex or whose hospitalizations turn out to be "complex" for any one of a myriad of reasons. Nurses' efforts are measured in hours worked or in the proportion of a full-time equivalent position occupied, regardless of credentials or experience. As a result, the same or identical ratios in different nursing units or in different hospitals may mean that patients are receiving very disparate "doses" of nursing time in relation to their needs. This will be the case particularly if unadjusted staffing levels across different types of hospitals (for profit, not for profit, specialized or comprehensive) or across very different types of nursing units are directly compared.

Furthermore, many staffing measures gloss over differences in needs for nursing care found across patients in a single unit on a specific shift (let alone the patients cared for in a unit over an extended period or across all the units in a hospital over a year). It is well-known that patients with the same medical diagnoses can require quite different amounts of nursing attention.[4] Consequently, most staffing measures tell us nothing about how well nursing time for specific patients is being adjusted to ensure that needs are being met. Again, staffing measures used in research are averages. They serve as general indicators of the scale of investments a hospital makes in nursing human resources, and provide limited data about the conditions under which specific patients are cared for.

The direct nursing care patients receive reflects decisions made by different parties at many levels in a health care system. The story of staffing is fundamentally one of "trickle-down" resource allocation. As decisions get closer to the point of care (to nurses' assignments on a particular shift), they become more visible to patients and nurses.

Payers from the public and private sectors in health care systems set rates they will pay institutions for providing hospital care. Executives and other leaders in hospitals make decisions allocating their financial resources across the various operating divisions in their institutions. Although human resource expenditures (and nursing personnel expenses) represent a major share of hospital budgets, they are not the only costs hospitals face and trade-offs must be made. Further allocation decisions apportion nursing personnel budgets to specific clinical service areas and to units within these services.

Still other decisions are made further downstream, with frontline managers at the nursing unit level and shift-level supervisors (such as house supervisors and charge nurses) making further smaller adjustments to nursing hours provided by different types of personnel over pay periods and shorter intervals. Supplemental staffing to deal with short-term contingencies, such as higher patient census levels or patients with unexpectedly complex needs, are commonly handled this way. Finally, once a frontline (bedside) clinician receives a patient load for a given shift, she or he makes a variety of decisions to prioritize and organize care for each patient and to budget time across the assigned patients. Minute-to-minute decisions about bedside care vary from nurse to nurse and are influenced by both experience on the job and expertise in working with a particular patient population. All of these decisions, from the upper reaches of the health care system down to the bedside, affect the care patients experience as well as patients' outcomes. Nevertheless, research on nurse staffing nearly always uses measures of resource allocation occurring at the top of health care organizations rather than ones made close to the bedside.

Measuring Outcomes

Slightly different challenges than those involved in measuring staffing come into play in measuring patient outcomes. Data sources for gauging the quality of health care are somewhat limited and researchers must balance data quality against costs in their studies.[5] Possible approaches include direct observation of care, which is intrusive and is generally better for examining process of care issues (such as the accurate administration of medications and consistent hand washing) than patient outcomes. Patients and health care workers can be surveyed, but such "soft" data have limited appeal to many stakeholders in health care. Data about perceptions and satisfaction often serve as a complement to "harder" objective data (such as risk-adjusted patient mortality statistics).

There are a fixed number of options for measuring patient health outcomes objectively. Understanding their possibilities and limitations provides a clear indication of why one particular source of data and one particular set of outcome variables have been used so heavily by researchers.

Health care providers leave a record of care they deliver in patients' charts. This could offer extensive opportunities to examine the care provided as well as the health status of patients at various stages of treatment, but the content of charts varies widely from institution to institution. Furthermore, the thoroughness and reliability of assessments can differ markedly from nurse to nurse and across the various clinicians from other disciplines. Much nursing care and many observations are never recorded in the patient's permanent health care record. Although the administration of medications is carefully tracked, for instance, other nursing actions are documented less systematically, including many forms of supportive care, such as comfort, hygiene, and safety measures. Nurses make many clinical observations that are not necessarily recorded on flow sheets and in charting, especially if the findings are within "normal" ranges. Nonetheless, the observations take time to make and interpret and influence the patient's clinical course. The comprehensive yet succinct charting that educators and hospital officials alike hope for is rarely seen in practice. As a result, data from patient charts are often of questionable reliability.

A further practical problem is the time and expense involved in sifting out important nursing-related variables from patient-care records. It can be very expensive to collect data about specific aspects of patients' care from charts, requiring many hours of trained abstractor time. In many health care systems, some key variables are routinely culled from hospital patients' charts (a process called abstraction) for record-keeping purposes, insurance billing, and often both. Discharge abstracts may reflect certain aspects of patients' clinical courses particularly well, especially when the accuracy of the data influences hospital reimbursement and funding. However, not all the data fields in discharge abstracts are equally reliable and high levels of certain negative outcomes that appear to be indicators of poor nursing care may actually reflect other factors (for instance, the conscientiousness of coders). Beyond the major reason for the patient's admission and whether he or she leaves the hospital dead or alive, the care taken to record the precise diagnoses and procedures and details about the patient's concurrent illnesses and complications is heavily determined by reimbursement rules (related, for instance, to the importance of precise coding of specific admission codes and comorbidities and complications). If hospitals decide that these differences justify investments in attentive coding, the accuracy of the relevant data fields will be that much better. Coding accuracy becomes particularly critical when attempting to conduct fair comparisons of outcomes across nursing units or hospitals that treat patients with different baseline risks of poor outcomes. Without sound, consistent information about comorbidities, high levels of poor outcomes might suggest that hospitals with clienteles of many chronically ill and elderly patients are providing inferior care when it may really indicate that they are providing sound treatment to a challenging patient population.

Because of the costliness and practical limitations of other data sources, despite their many disadvantages databases of discharge abstracts assembled for administrative purposes provide most of the information about the outcomes of hospital care used in nurse staffing research. Researchers continue to place a great deal of emphasis on complications in hospital care (particularly surgical complications) and have examined falls and pressure ulcers as theoretically responsive to nurse staffing levels, even though the quality of routine documentation of these events can be quite poor. Various surveillance protocols for identifying clinical problems such as falls or infections that include chart reviews in addition to other data sources (such as other hospital information systems) are sometimes implemented.

The specific patient outcomes that are examined are similarly constrained. Choices generally fall into two types of indicators: complications and mortality. Complications are patient conditions that are not present on admission and develop during treatment including pressure ulcers and wound infections. Some complications are believed to be influenced by nurses' actions, and researchers have proposed that they are potential indicators of the quality of nursing care. However, in addition to the question of the consistency of the recording of complications, the sensitivity of the occurrence of complications to differences in the quality of nursing care has been the subject of intense debate. Postoperative respiratory infections and pulmonary emboli are examples of complications that are purportedly sensitive to nursing care, but there are clearly patient characteristics, such as age- and condition-related factors, that influence patients' risks for developing them. Overall, there is much reason to be skeptical about the measurement of complications and their use in outcomes research.[6] Because it may better capture quality of care, failure to rescue, a hybrid measure that examines deaths following complications, has been proposed as a potential alternative.[7] It has been suggested that failure to rescue is influenced by the human and material resources available in an institution for timely recognition of serious patient-care problems and rapid initiation of appropriate treatment, aspects of nursing care not necessarily reflected in complication rates.

Mortality rates among specific patient clienteles in a hospital have long been popular outcomes variables in hospital outcomes research. Despite their shortcomings as indicators of hospital quality, they are still commonly used by staffing researchers. The underlying assumption is that poor nurse staffing heightens the risk of serious errors of commission and omission in care and leads to higher mortality rates than normal. Researchers analyze death rates less out of a belief that they are particularly sensitive to differences in nursing care and more because reliable data on other patient outcomes are difficult, if not impossible, to obtain economically on a sufficient scale to conduct outcomes research.

Historically, scholars in nursing have objected to the narrowness of mortality as an outcome, preferring the broader perspective on human health offered by concepts such as psychosocial well-being and functional status.

They have also raised valid questions about the sensitivity of mortality to nursing care. Nurses are not the only professionals whose judgments and actions can prevent patient deaths. Additionally, many of the actions that nurses take that influence mortality rates in hospitals fall within the "interdependent" scope of practice shared with medicine and other disciplines, rather than the independent practice parameters that nurses take most or all responsibility for.

On a practical level, death in hospitals for most subgroups of patients is fortunately relatively rare. Systematically detecting and identifying abnormally high mortality rates suggestive of clinically significant problems in quality of care can require reviewing many thousands of cases. However, patient deaths have an unequivocal meaning and can be easily identified in many databases and therefore will most likely continue to be studied until data sources that offer opportunities to examine broader classes of patient outcomes can be identified and harnessed.

Selecting which patients outcomes will be examined is another recurring problem. Patients differ in the outcomes that are meaningful indicators of the quality of care they receive. For instance, death in patients in end-stage organ failure or with terminal cancer does not have the same meaning as death in relatively young, healthy patients undergoing elective surgeries. Patient groups also differ in their likelihood of experiencing good or poor outcomes (for instance, patients undergoing bone marrow transplantation face very different risks than women admitted for childbirth). Even within a pool of patients admitted to the same institution for a similar diagnosis or procedure, risks for untoward outcomes may differ widely depending on age, comorbid conditions, and disease stage.

Examining narrowly defined patient groups raises concerns about the generalizability of findings, such as whether findings about relationships between staffing and outcomes for patients undergoing specialized surgeries apply to hospitalized patients at large. However, measuring outcomes in very broad clienteles often raises questions about the relevance and/or sensitivity of the measures across all the types of patients being studied. Patient falls occur at very different rates and have different causes and implications for in-patient geriatric medicine units than in labor and delivery units, for instance.

Clearly, unit-specific staffing measures and outcome measures tailored to the specific clienteles cared for in those units would be best. This has rarely been achieved. One notable exception was a large and complex study of the outcomes of in-patient AIDS care involving forty units from twenty hospitals across the United States. Carried out in the early 1990s, it involved carefully collected unit-level data and a battery of tailored measures from nurses and patients that ranged from nurse burnout to patient mortality.[8] Since then researchers and nurse managers and executives have begun to make serious headway in assembling data sets with detailed staffing information about patient-care units.[9] Work by a number of data consortiums, for instance the National Database of Nursing Quality Indicators sponsored by the American Nurses Association,[10] is moving in this direction. However, some basic measurement issues have yet to be resolved. For instance, patient falls and pressure ulcers are commonly used as unit-specific outcome measures in this work and adjustments for unit-to-unit differences in inherent patient risk in the patient populations in single units over time have yet to be perfected and consistently applied for even these outcomes. It should also be noted that outcomes measures sensitive to unit-level staffing differences have yet to be developed for most specialties in nursing.

Fortunately, the search for meaningful patient outcomes suitable for staffing research continues. A host of instruments believed to be potentially sensitive to nursing care have been developed and cataloged.[11] However, many of these indicators were designed for research on special nursing treatments. It is not always clear how they could or should be used in large-scale observational research because studying the quality of nursing care routinely delivered on the front lines of nursing units and community settings is a distinctly different exercise from conducting randomized trials of nursing interventions. Even when newer measurements with plausible connections to nursing in hospital care are available, they may be so cumbersome and expensive to use that it is impractical to employ them in studies with enough subjects and data collection points to study the impacts of staffing.

A major dilemma faced by staffing researchers is that outcome measures must often be collected over and above the clinical work going on in care settings, often at considerable inconvenience and expense. In the words of Dennis O'Leary, the president of the Joint Commission on Accreditation of Healthcare Organizations (the largest health care accreditation body in the United States), "Performance measurement will be a sham until data are collected as by-products of care delivery, a capability that only the Electronic Medical Record (EMR) can provide." Awaiting better data sources and measures, we must accept trade-offs of quantity for quality of data and recognize that because of limitations in available data, researchers have not yet captured the full impact of staffing on patient outcomes.

The "Black Box"—Process of Care

Plausible explanations for the effects of staffing on nursing-sensitive outcomes must ultimately cite or infer differences in the nursing care patients receive under varying staffing conditions. Interestingly, however, the connections between staffing and bedside care (or the "black box" of mechanisms through which staffing levels affect patient outcomes) remain largely unexplored territory. There is an implicit assumption that staffing variations lead to quantitative and qualitative differences in the nursing care patients receive and that some of these differences influence the likelihood of various outcomes. However, a better understanding of the mechanisms involved is critical to administrators, policymakers, and clinicians seeking to make better decisions about how to allocate staffing.

The assessments and judgments that nurses use to shape the way they work with patients do not always easily map onto the medical diagnoses that bring patients into treatment.[12] Furthermore, existing taxonomies of nursing diagnoses, interventions, and outcomes have serious limitations and have not yet been widely enough adopted to enable much progress in documenting the process of nursing care.[13] Standardized approaches to data collection that examine the process of care at the bedside and are suitable for either routine use or large-scale data collection do not yet exist.

Overall, for lack of data sources, research that could facilitate better decision making about staffing and allocation of other resources has not yet begun. Managers and policymakers have little sense of whether adjusting staffing or adjusting other factors in hospitals (or adjusting both types of variables in different proportions) will produce the types of patient outcomes they want.

Fleshing out the "black box" may also foster the development of theoretical coherence in this literature by helping to explain why so many research studies find support for only a fraction of the expected significant associations between staffing and outcomes. For instance, in large data sets across multiple states in the United States, Christine Kovner and her colleagues found an association between nurse staffing and only one of the four postsurgical outcomes they examined, postoperative pneumonia.[14] Jack Needleman and his colleagues found that only six (of eleven) and two (of fourteen) outcomes they examined for medical and surgical patients, respectively, showed associations with staffing.[15] Although few in health care believe that nursing care is implicated in every type of adverse patient outcome, no one knows which negative findings reflect the lack of a significant influence of nursing on specific outcomes and which findings reflect statistical and methodological artifact. Does a failure to find a connection between staffing levels and urinary tract infections in every study mean that urinary tract infections are not significantly influenced by nursing care? Or is there some issue with measurement or sampling in these studies causing a staffing-outcomes association to appear on some occasions and not others? A quantitative understanding of what nurses do, practically speaking, can only help clarify such issues and lead to overarching theoretical connections in this area of research.

In summary, explaining the connections between staffing and outcomes has been hampered by limitations in measures and data collection approaches. Understanding how staffing affects quality of care at the bedside will be markedly assisted by the widespread introduction of the Electronic Medical Record. When nurses' interventions and patients' responses to them are routinely documented in the course of delivering care, research possibilities will expand dramatically. Although such future research at the "micro" level of care delivery will consume a great deal of effort, it will almost certainly prove immensely rewarding.

The Nature of Staffing Research

Nothing in the preceding comments is intended to undercut the contributions of the articles currently in this literature. Furthermore, nothing here should be construed as implying that action should wait for further research data to become available. Are the data linking staffing with outcomes sufficient to influence managerial practice and public policy? Absolutely. It is common sense that there is a maximum number of patients that any given nurse can manage under a set of defined circumstances. It is also self-evident that this number needs to be adjusted downward as the complexity and instability of patients' conditions increases. The results of staffing research are consistent with what nurses and others have instinctively believed and experienced for many years. It is in some ways surprising that empirical support for these ideas was so long in coming. However, those who apply and cite staffing research, especially in policy contexts, must be clear about which parts of their arguments about regulating staffing are drawn from research studies, which contentions reflect other data sources, and which portions are merely statements of their values and personal beliefs.[16] For instance, this literature does not and cannot provide incontrovertible evidence that specific staffing levels at the bedside in particular types of nursing units are safe or unsafe. There are simply too many unsettled issues in measuring staffing and patient outcomes and too few findings that explain why staffing-outcomes connections occur to make such direct statements and extrapolations.

The data in this literature so far have been based on observational, not experimental, studies. One of the first rules of research methodology is, of course, that a correlation between two variables does not necessarily mean that one factor directly causes the other. Reasonable explanations for correlations can go in either direction. If variables A and B are correlated, A may cause B, B may cause A, or a third variable associated with both of the original two variables can be the "true" reason for the connection. For instance, assume for the purposes of illustration that high potato chip consumption is associated with lower secondary school grades. The explanation is not necessarily that eating more potato chips causes poorer academic performance, although one can surely come up with a compelling, if scientifically questionable, story about the effects of heavy doses of salt, fat, and starch on the brain. Students with poor academic performance may seek solace in potato chips or a third factor (such as heavy television watching engaged in by major potato chip consumers that tends to limit study time) may be one of the "real" connecting factors.

Any demonstrated effect on patient safety outcomes requires careful investigation. For instance, a correlation between staffing and patient safety may be an effect of nurses choosing not to work in hospitals that have reputations for patient safety problems, rather than patient safety being a direct consequence of high or low staffing levels per se. Staffing could be associated with other characteristics of hospitals or their patients the way television watching connects junk food and bad grades, and some or all of these "other" factors may be directly responsible for patient safety outcomes. Staffing in better-equipped hospitals or those with better qualified physicians may be higher and these and other such variables might account for some or all of the association between staffing and outcomes. Researchers handle this by controlling for as many characteristics of patients and providers as possible in the statistical models. Nonetheless, whether there are factors that vary alongside staffing that could account for part or all of its effects or modify its impacts on different patients under different circumstances is still not completely clear.

The generalizability of the staffing effects identified so far remains an open question. The findings of these studies are derived from statistical models that depict connections between variables in particular data sets. They represent stylized portraits of patterns in data, with the rough edges sanded off, not only because the staffing and outcomes variables are approximations but because modeling requires making a host of assumptions about the data being analyzed and the nature of the relationships between variables. As a result, the studies establish that in specific data sets, for specific subgroups of hospitalized patients, the frequency of certain outcomes has been statistically associated with staffing levels. The only defensible conclusion possible for most studies is that when average staffing levels are high, average patient outcomes tend to be better.

Staffing researchers make good-faith efforts to be transparent about methods and assumptions. However, the results are always, at best, an approximation or an attempt to portray what is going on in a specific data set, with no guarantees about whether the findings apply elsewhere. In the often quoted words of the statistician George Box, "All models are wrong, but some are useful."[17] Researchers, journal editors, and users of this research certainly hope that results apply beyond the specific institutions and points in time that are studied. However, after some basic conditions are met, it's very difficult to know one way or another whether the effects occur in other contexts. We simply do not know how real-world differences in hospitals, nurses, and patients affect the applicability of the findings. The authors of a recent statistical handbook suggest that we "treat every model as tentative, [and] best described . . . as subject to change without notice."[18] As a result, all research results based on statistical modeling should be extrapolated with caution; readers of the staffing literature need to be particularly sensitive to this caveat.

Replication, refinement, and extension of the findings now in the literature are all necessary. Overall, however, a point of diminishing returns is rapidly approaching with currently favored modeling approaches and readily available data sources. The overall finding of the extant staffing literature—that certain outcomes and staffing appear to move together when viewed at a distance from bedside care—is unlikely to be altered by more research of the same kind. Staffing researchers are still grasping at the shadow and must now turn to new data sources and research approaches in order to capture the substance of nursing in their work.

Opportunities and Risks for the Nursing Profession

The wide and intense interest in this research is due in large part to the deepening nurse shortage facing most Western countries. Much public attention has been focused on this issue and nurses have been emboldened and empowered by evidence that their numbers within health care institutions make a difference. Many observers believe that staffing research provides a glimpse of the types of patient outcomes that can be expected to deteriorate as staffing shortages worsen. Of course, projections of this sort place a great deal of confidence in existing research findings. Furthermore, such forecasts also assume that demographic projections for the nurse workforce and the general population are correct, that health care systems will continue to employ nurses in similar roles, and no other major changes affecting the supply of or demand for nurses will occur. Even if we read these findings and trends with a skeptical eye, coming shortfalls in the nurse workforce will cause problems with the quality of care in at least some institutions, and perhaps across entire communities and nations. So given this body of studies and the health care context, where should research, policy, and development of the profession proceed next?[19]

Gauging the Contributions of Frontline Human Services Work

The crisis in nursing can be interpreted in the context of much broader problems in the delivery of human services in many Western countries. Many communities in the United States face recurring shortages of frontline human service workers, such as social service caseworkers, elementary and secondary school teachers, police officers, and nurses.

Low remuneration for many of these workers plays a role in these shortages. There is a basic public policy issue intertwined with the value placed on this type of hands-on work by pay rates. Although there are exceptions, many service workers are paid to "cover" clients in locations over time, rather than to provide specific easily demarcated services to individuals, as physicians and attorneys do, for instance. The measurement of the work is difficult. There may be many routines or tasks perceived as uncomplicated and unimportant. To an outside eye, taking on an additional one or two or five clients, communities, or activities might appear to make little difference. There are questions in the minds of many about how much education and skill is really involved in these types of work, as well as whether the role of the workers in producing good or bad outcomes is sufficient to justify increasing pay, preparation, or both. Overall, there is resistance to paying more, often with higher taxes, for the services. Yet bitter complaints ensue when the services fall short, for instance when waiting times become too long or when service is perceived as being ineffective or insensitive.

Research studies are in the forefront of discussions inside and outside the profession about how to manage an expensive and increasingly scarce resource such as nursing and somewhat less prominent in discussions of how best to manage medical care. (Nonetheless, some health-outcomes research dealing with physician care has become part of policy discussions, including studies on the outcomes of patients with board-certified physicians as well as physicians with more experience in treating specific illnesses or performing certain surgeries.) It might prove instructive to compare medical and nursing care in terms of the nature of the work, the patient's experience of it, the nature of research that examines it, and the implications of all these factors for decision making about the allocation of resources.

There are striking differences in the nature of the services provided by physicians and generalist nurses (those who are not advanced practice nurses). In the paradigm of medical care, patients see clinicians at specific points in time to identify or diagnose specific clinical problems so that acceptable treatment approaches can be selected. There are well-defined decision points in the process of delivering medical care. An entire methodological tradition, clinical epidemiology, is essentially an arsenal of techniques for validating diagnostic maneuvers and evaluating treatment approaches in medicine. Outcomes research within clinical epidemiology aims to identify the variations in patient and provider characteristics and in the environment of care that influence the outcomes of specific types of medical care.

Think about the public's experience of medical care. The stories that people tell about health care involve the miracles of medical diagnosis (the causes of mysterious ailments unveiled) and of medical treatment (heroic triumphs of science over nature run amok in our bodies). The structure of the work, the research enterprise involved in institutionalizing and improving it, and the public understanding of it are closely aligned and contribute to its status. The economic rewards involved in practicing medicine were clearer when physicians were generously paid (by the medical act rendered) for providing highly specific professional services. In the United States, reimbursement rates increasingly are being scaled down, physicians receive a salary rather than being paid per patient encounter, and there are increased pressures to allow nonspecialist physicians and even nonphysicians to deliver some medical services. These changes are producing a great deal of discomfort and discontent because they downplay the uniqueness of physicians' qualifications and judgments and involve regulating the conditions of practice more than ever before. The conditions of medical practice are now coming to closely resemble those of nursing work, and the intense unhappiness seen among physicians should come as little surprise.[20]

Nursing care, as it is delivered by most frontline clinicians, has a different consistency or "feel" than medical treatment. There are indeed specific "diagnosis" and "treatment" decisions in nursing practice (although they are not necessarily best labeled as such, given the blurred sense of those terms from their use in the medical paradigm). Nurses make perhaps a hundred or more of these judgments during a typical workday, but the decisions themselves are generally not the immediate reasons patients become recipients of nursing care. Many nurses' decisions occur while implementing treatment plans developed by other clinicians. The thought processes involved in some nursing acts, such as patient positioning, mouth care, and so forth, may be interpreted as being so trivial (at least to the untrained eye) as to make their study ridiculous. There are few well-established research approaches for examining and evaluating nurses' practice decisions. Furthermore, whereas intense research activity in medicine is devoted to developing and testing interventions for use at the front lines of patient- care delivery, comparatively little attention in nursing research is devoted to direct bedside care. Even though front-line illness care is the type of work most nurses are engaged in, academic nursing has all but turned away from studying it. Much research in nursing examines aspects of health not normally handled by the bedside generalist nurse and expanded roles or practice settings for nurses. Most bedside nursing work is not easily measured using available data sources and therefore is not especially well researched (which also militates against its being considered knowledge work).

Most theoretical work in nursing must be interpreted very broadly to address the work of bedside nurses. Sometimes it is nearly impossible to draw a connection between the generalist role and nursing theory. Some may argue that institutional leaders are as responsible as scholars for the failure to widely adopt discipline-specific theories and frameworks in practice settings, but the result is the same: theoretical work in nursing is rarely applied to the majority of problems that concern clinicians in the field. Nonetheless, in the eyes of academics and academically trained nurses, the role of nursing is clear if not always visible: nurses work on a practical level with the physiological and psychological needs that accompany illnesses and life transitions and their associated medical treatments.[21]

As experienced by the public, nursing care is the backdrop against which the "magic" of diagnosis and treatment in hospitals unfolds. Stories of nursing care and the gratitude of patients for it are less the stories of triumphs than of living through hardships. Much nursing care consists of acts needed to endure crises rather than resolve them. The care itself and the issues nurses deal with (pain, fear, physical incapacity, complexity, and risks presented by drugs and equipment needed for treatment) are reminders of the vulnerabilities in the human condition. Until individuals are confronted with the need for nursing care, many are unaware of the knowledge and skill involved in managing all of these elements. The public trusts nurses and believe that nurses have altruistic motives. This is clear at least in the United States, where annual surveys rank nurses as the most ethical and honest workers. However, laypeople's understanding of what nurses actually do is often limited. Although some simply don't want to hear about the grittier aspects of nurses' work, more seem to share nurses' perceptions that they are ordinary people doing an unglamorous and sometimes very difficult job. The shadowy understanding of nursing work outside the profession is worsened by nurses' modesty and tendency to remain silent about their practices and talk only about their caring and compassion.

Additionally, although nurses understand the need for rigorous basic and continuing education as well as the role of experience in ensuring proficient nursing care, the importance of education and specialization are not always clear outside the profession. Many members of the public and even the policy community believe that the most important prerequisites for being a good nurse are a strong back, a strong stomach, and a good heart. The brain power necessary to do the work may get left out of the equation. The notion that bedside nursing doesn't require much advanced education has been a staple of one side of the discussions about local, state, and national resource allocation in nursing over the years. The MD degree and parallel credentials in other countries have well-understood meanings as entry points to medical practice that nursing degrees do not, especially because multiple entry levels for nursing persist. Arguably, the lack of a uniform educational level for entry to nursing practice in many countries and protracted infighting within the profession around educational issues do not help the situation. The situation with nursing education in many countries, notably the United States, is befuddling to nurses from all quarters to say nothing of the general public.

Overall, frontline nursing work suffers from invisibility both within and outside the profession. Whether invisibility is a cause or an effect of the way nurses are paid for their work is unclear, but it plays a role in the broader problems faced in reform. It is difficult to measure nursing time in a reliable and meaningful way that allows for fair cost accounting. It is easier not to think of the nursing care of each patient individually but rather to bundle care as "nursing services," consider these services as a cost center, and provide incentives to reduce expenditures on them as much as possible. Depending on whose stance one takes or what time frame one looks at, it may be more "cost effective" to spend less on nurse staffing and suffer the consequences in turnover and perhaps patient safety problems than to make investments in nursing personnel beyond certain minimums. The tendency to think of nursing this way is accentuated by escalating demands to control operating costs in health care.

Staffing research helped immensely in making nursing services visible to the public. That patient mortality in hospitals was linked to nurse staffing levels at all came as a wake-up call to many. Many readers also inferred that these studies indicated that nursing care itself was an important contributor to patient outcomes, even if care was not directly measured in these studies.

Nonetheless, better allocation of staffing must be driven by a more nuanced understanding of clinical acts and decisions than can be gained with existing tools. If the process and outcomes of care at the bedside, the judgment components of nursing work, and the organizational conditions needed to perform such knowledge work do not soon become part of the research discourse , the types of findings researchers generate will continue to drive leadership and policy decisions that fall short in the long run. Attention to these elements must begin inside nursing. We must care about what occurs at the bedside on a scholarly level within the profession before we can put forward compelling arguments to those outside it that will help ensure high-quality nursing care.

The Dangers in a Narrow Reading of Staffing Research

A focus on finding pairs of hands without attending to what nurses do to influence various outcomes and to qualitative differences in how nurses with different backgrounds and experience levels deliver nursing care may well prove counterproductive. It is unlikely that staffing numbers alone are the sole determinant of patient safety. Raising staffing levels may not have the desired effects if the nursing personnel being added are not well equipped to deliver the types of care that are needed. Furthermore, if it is true that well-educated and experienced nurses cannot deliver high quality care in poorly managed environments, then if managers don't construct or reconstruct favorable conditions for practice, increases in staffing without safeguards or improvements for practice conditions may not translate into better outcomes either. There is evidence that practice environment conditions other than staffing may explain variations in important nurse and patient outcomes in hospitals.[22]

Nurse executives and managers know intuitively that the relationships between staffing and outcomes are quite complex. The staffing decisions that most managers regularly make are intended to respond to differences in needs for care across patient populations. Research that more clearly identifies the mechanisms responsible for good and poor patient outcomes under different staffing conditions will probably suggest more subtle interventions than uniform increases in staffing levels alone.

A major policy initiative that has been the subject of intense discussion internationally involves mandated minimum nurse-to-patient ratios.[23] The intent of staffing ratio legislation is to protect patient safety and encourage those driven away by poor working conditions to enter or return to hospital practice. The safety or advisability of imposing minimum ratios cannot directly be inferred from the research literature.[24] Although the stated purpose of minimum ratios is to prevent institutions from lowering staffing to levels at which safe care is impossible, mandated staffing ratios can also interfere with the ability of staff and managers to modify staffing levels or change ratios according to patient needs and available staff. There is nothing that prevents agencies from adjusting staffing upward from mandated minimums. However, to afford prescribed levels of nurse-to-patient ratios around the clock (which may not always serve patient needs), hospitals can be forced to shift resources away from salaried positions and hours worked by certain types of personnel not monitored by the legislation but whose work can greatly benefit patients (such as dedicated institution-wide teams for certain types of care such as lifting patients or intravenous therapy, or for unlicensed assistive personnel). A balance has to be struck between protecting the public from the dangers of low staffing levels and eliminating too many of the degrees of freedom available to responsible managers in designing staffing plans that do, in fact, benefit both patient safety and the bottom line, and allow for meaningful, satisfying work for nurses.

There are yet other reasons to think carefully about the complex set of factors, including but not limited to staffing levels, involved in patient safety. It is important to clarify the difference between staffing problems and deficiencies in practice, for instance. Although low staffing levels put constraints on the comprehensiveness and quality of nursing that patients receive, care that falls short of accepted practice standards is found across the entire range of staffing found in hospitals. Quality monitoring and improvement are essential activities in hospitals. Diverting resources away from the oversight of care by managers and administrators, which was a major strategy in hospital reengineering in the 1990s, can be very unwise. There can be severe long-term consequences of cutting positions dedicated to career development for clinicians and enhancing bedside care, like those of clinical specialists and educators. Patient safety disasters can and do occur in the presence of objectively "acceptable" staffing levels where nursing practice is unmonitored and unsafe conditions are not corrected. Problematic staff communication and deficiencies in staff education (as well as staffing problems) repeatedly lead the lists of identified root causes of sentinel events (serious errors leading to patient injury or death) reported to the Joint Commission on Accreditation of Healthcare Organizations in the United States.[25]

An overly narrow reading of staffing research could feed into deskilling initiatives in nursing service and education. As the expression goes, "People will do what you inspect, not what you expect." Although the gravest threat for the public is that there will not be enough attentive, skillful nursing care to go around, a focus on crude staffing ratios could lead to much energy being directed into either changing or challenging the levels being set and the metrics for measuring staffing, instead of solving fundamental quality-of-care problems. If numbers of nurses alone are of sole concern, various standards in nursing education may be challenged as impediments to the quick and inexpensive production of an adequate supply of nurses. Nurse educators may feel considerable pressure from outside the profession to shorten training programs by eliminating experiences that are costly and scarce and can become rate-limiting steps in graduating new nurses. Service agencies could hold to the very minimum qualifications, training, and experience levels that regulators require or that research suggests are related to safety, even when common sense would suggest that higher levels would be in patients' interests.

There could be incentives for leaders to engineer short-term improvements in staffing statistics for their institutions and communities while letting opportunities for long-term stabilization of the nurse workforce slip away. Indeed, the unprecedented combination of stagnant growth and increasing retirements in the nurse workforce coupled with an increasing demand for health services among aging populations in Western countries requires a fundamental rethinking of existing approaches to preparing nurses, deploying their labor, and managing their practice environments. Focusing entirely on solutions such as importing nurses from other countries and increasing the production of new nurses without attending to long-term problems in the realities of nursing work could have disastrous consequences.

Directions for the Profession

Staffing research and the debate about staffing ratios have generated renewed scholarly interest in the work of frontline generalist nurses. For a variety of reasons, research on bedside nursing has not been fashionable. Nurse scholars, especially those educated at the doctoral level, often come to regard day-to-day practice issues as undeserving of focused attention. Some feel that examining bedside practice is too close to the notion of nurses studying themselves to represent a serious scholarly endeavor. Still others believe that nurse researchers should assist in constructing the world of practice as it should be by developing an evidence base for the future roles of nurses, rather than describing the world of practice as it exists, burdened as it is with difficult entanglements with other disciplines and long standing image problems. It could also be argued that many nurse academics "go native" and adopt the priorities of university life and move away from the perspectives and sensitivities of the bedside nurse. In any case, the rejection of bedside practice by academe reflects tensions that go in both directions. The disdain of many practicing nurses for academic pursuits and scholarly reflection can be extreme, with academic research being considered arcane, insular, self-perpetuating, and even useless by many bedside clinicians.

Staffing-outcomes research is building bridges across this divide by returning scholarly focus to the profession's roots and to the work of its rank and file. It is also stimulating a resurgence of interest in nursing research across the entire profession. It is essential that nurse scholars ensure that efforts to date serve as a beginning rather than an endpoint in a renewed research focus on the clinical mission in in-patient care.

Nursing has moved from a field with a very small research base to being a profession that has invested huge amounts of human and material resources in the research enterprise. It now heavily socializes its members to value research data. The relationship between nurse staffing and outcomes has moved from the status of firmly held conjecture and is well on its way to being empirically demonstrated in ways that will make health care better and safer.

However, we need to remember that not all questions can be resolved with empirical data and that not all of the outcomes that nurses influence will be readily documented, now or in the future. We should beware of a misplaced faith in research alone to drive responsible resource allocation. Empirical findings are a starting point, but ultimately there will never be enough data that pinpoint the effects of specific choices with enough certainty to eliminate the need for clearly articulated values and a willingness to act on them.

Nurses come to work prepared to be busy, to earn their pay, and to uphold the trust that the public places in them, and health care managers understand their role as stewards of their institutions' resources as well as overseers of public safety. A healthy respect for the elements of nursing that cannot be quantified is needed. Optimizing outcomes requires that everyone involved in hospital care respect the spirit as well as the letter of regulations and guidelines. Without firm numbers about the staffing levels at which risks to patients become unacceptable (and even with such figures), it is an act of faith to embrace models of care that provide a critical mass of professional nurses to handle patients' needs and the risks they face. It is an act of faith to staff institutions in such a manner that nurses do not find themselves in constant motion over an eight- or twelve-hour period day after day without maneuvering room to deal with unexpected events. Ensuring that nurses have resource specialists who can help them keep their practice current and safe and move them forward at every stage in their development as clinicians is also a gesture of faith and respect for practice.

Grounding decisions in principles such as these takes certain ideas for granted. Specifically, it assumes nursing is knowledge work that demands time for reflection—that it involves thinking as well as doing. It requires an understanding that nurses cannot deal effectively with patients if they are constantly under stress. The term "faith" seems particularly apt because such choices force nurses in leadership roles at all levels in the profession to hold to their convictions in the face of heavy pressures from above and below to proceed in other directions. Recognizing these complexities also requires activists inside and outside unions who fight for staffing ratios to realize that rigid application of ratios may be counterproductive and may actually lead to losing the substance of nursing.

The full range of benefits from allocating nurse human resources above operational minimums may never be definitively documented. Given the limitations of empirical research, we may need to content ourselves with justifying some investments in nurse human resources as simply the "right" things to do from the point of view of human relations and social responsibility.

A last point about the use of staffing research in the development of the profession bears mention. If we accord a privileged place to research evidence, we must be prepared for the eventuality that sometimes research will not support popular strategies for employing nurses. For example, under some circumstances high staffing levels may be ineffective or even dangerous. An interesting example of staffing and outcomes data that were interpreted this way is found in work by Callaghan and colleagues.[26] In a study that incorporated careful controls for patient characteristics, these authors found that higher nurse staffing levels were associated with higher mortality levels in a cohort of very low birth-weight infants. They hypothesized that higher staffing levels might lead to increased handling of these fragile infants, with heightened risks for infection, among other clinical problems. For some clinical populations, staffing mixes that include non-professional nursing staff may prove as safe and effective, if not more so, as staffing models consisting entirely of professional nurses. Although identifying and holding firm to values is extremely important, if as nurses we have any faith in empiricism we must be willing to move from our beliefs if facts point us in new directions.

As nurses and nursing attempt to uphold their end of the agreement with the public to provide essential health care services, it is vital that empirical research on nurses' work and the conditions that influence its outcomes continues. Some of the complexities of staffing research have been discussed at length here, along with a plea for attention to the effects of staffing at the point of care. Ultimately, however, the limitations and uncertainties common to research of any kind will always need to be considered before translating the results of staffing-outcomes studies. At best, those who fail to stay within the boundaries of what can be reasonably surmised from specific studies when citing them risk damaging their credibility, when well-articulated arguments correctly citing research data in context could be just as effective. At worst, harm to patients can occur when conclusions based on misinterpreted data are applied in practice. In the end, as we reinvent the nursing profession in the coming decades, a clear sense of our values, an understanding of other stakeholders' interests, and a willingness to take well-calculated risks will all guide the future every bit as much as research data.

Conclusion

Nurses Wanted: Sentimental Men and Women Need Not Apply

Sioban Nelson and Suzanne Gordon

As editors of this collection we set ourselves a single goal: to alert our colleagues and collaborators to the problems caused by the current discussion of caring in nursing and its impact on the way nursing practice is constructed. We confronted this endeavor with a great deal of trepidation, wary lest some think we were arguing for the abandonment of care. This collection attempts to walk that fine line between valuing the caring work nursing provides and calling on nurses to think about and talk about their work in new, more accurate, and thus more helpful, ways. It also expresses concern about the way health care cost-cutting is transforming nursing practice, sometimes with the assent of nurses themselves.

In the early days of nursing's professionalization in the nineteenth century, nurse reformers from the battlefields of Florence Nightingale's Crimea to the American Civil War publicly lamented the romantic fashion that led thousands of women to flood into nursing. The kind of women needed on those battlefields or in the wards of the new medicalized hospitals were not the doe-eyed soft-hearted women of romantic fiction. Clever, hard-working, tough-minded women were what was needed.

Today the same kind of tough-minded individuals are needed, if we are to have enough qualified nurses now and in the future. Sentimentalizing about the joys of care and the relational aspects of nursing work in recruitment campaigns and in the plethora of other discourses on nursing will backfire on the hospital floor, when sweet-natured young men and women

Sentimental Women Need Not Apply, the famous quote from a Civil War advertisement, was the title of a 1988 film by Lawrence Hott and Diane Gray on the history of American nursing.

are thrown into the lion's den of the clinical world. Many new nursing recruits who enter the hospital universe leave the profession after only a couple of years. In a study reported in the U.S. health-policy journal *Health Affairs*, University of Pennsylvania nursing researcher Julie Sochalski found that in 2000 "a surprising 25 percent of new nurses employed in other fields, both men and women, said they had never worked in nursing. . . . In fact, 57 percent of new nurses working outside of nursing in 1996 had no experience in nursing." Of new nurses, men were leaving nursing at twice the rate of women.[1]

Anecdotally, nurses report that they find the hospital environment utterly inhospitable. What is interesting is why many of these new recruits are voting with their feet rather than engaging in the kind of political battles that will help them change the workplace. As some nurses tell us, their reluctance is a direct result of the script that drew them into the profession and the unrealistic expectations they had been led to have. When Gordon recently talked to several young nursing students at a conference of the Swiss Nurses Association, one of the feistiest and most political in the world, the students were both exhilarated and discouraged. They were optimistic about their ability to work for a political transformation of the nursing workforce but pessimistic because so few of their fellow students were interested in engaging in political work. "They've been attracted by conventional images of caring," the students said. "They think politics and caring are antithetical; they don't want to dirty their hands with the nitty-gritty of political activity."

The virtue script that we discuss also conceals realities about nursing work that have little to do with contemporary cost-cutting. Despite the angels, hearts, and hands, nursing is not for the fainthearted. Just as in the nineteenth century the same is true today—"Nurses Wanted: Sentimental Women Need Not Apply"—except today it applies to men as well! The narrow caring discourse that prevails today conceals the hard facts of nursing work. Nurses do things that hurt people: they drag people out of bed when they would much prefer to be left lying alone; they get people to do rehabilitation exercises when they feel like giving up; they change dressings on painful wounds; and they give patients information about their conditions that they would rather not learn. Sometimes their reward—as many contemporary campaigns trumpet—is indeed the gratitude in patients' eyes. But sometimes those eyes are full of anger, hostility, and sheer ingratitude. If people, as Beverly Malone and the U.S. National Student Nurses Association recruitment video suggest, are looking for a profession where "people love me," is nursing the profession they should choose?

We believe that the image the profession delivers to those it is trying to recruit and the iconography that is used to draw people toward the profession must do more than highlight moments of glorious success and human connection. Somehow it must prepare would-be nurses for the fact that much of their work will be with people who are in pain, frightened, anxious, and suffering and who do not want to and may not be able to connect on an emotional basis. Achieving this is tricky. It requires a fine balance between turning people on and turning people away—but it can be done.

Recently the Swiss Nurses Association dedicated 2005 as the year of visibility of nursing. Each cantonal chapter of the association launched a visibility project. While the chapters made caring visible, they went far beyond the traditional caring script and explored the entire range of activities that nurses engage in. One group produced a poster that showed what nurses do on an hourly basis every day. The clever graphics showed how much time nurses devote to technical and medical activities and to the skills involved in the kinds of basic bodily care that Aranda and Brown want nurses to preserve. Another group invited a senator, who is also the head of a health insurance fund, to follow a nurse at work. When the influential politician was finished tracking the nurse, he exclaimed that now he understood why the association had insisted on connecting talking and doing—the technical, emotional, and medical.

Although this book is not intended as a how-to guide, we believe that throughout the chapters the authors present guidance about what actions to take, what words and images to use to better illuminate the work and activities of nursing. In chapter one Suzanne Gordon's rewrite of one of the messages a nurse delivered in the Johnson & Johnson campaign illustrates how one can use the same number of words to convey very different messages. In the ad we reproduce from the British Columbia Nurses Union, we show how words and images can be cleverly combined to turn traditional stereotypes about nursing on their head.

We believe nurses should take a much more active role in rethinking how they describe their work. This is discussed at more length in Bernice Buresh and Suzanne Gordon's second edition of *From Silence to Voice: What Nurses Know and Must Communicate to the Public* (2006), also published in this series by Cornell University Press. We also believe they should carefully consider how their professional organizations and institutional employers depict them both in words and images. One has only to walk the halls of hospitals all over the world, or peruse the exhibitions hospitals and other employers mount as they try to recruit nurses, to see how easily the image of nursing could change if nurses took an active role in changing it.

Today, when we explore how hospitals depict nursing, what we notice is an endless series of smiling, sweet, virtuous-looking nurses decorating posters in hospital corridors or recruitment videos and exhibits. Next to them are photographs of physicians. The physicians (male and female) are invariably pictured with their arms folded across their chests, a hint of a smile perhaps, but usually with a serious look, accompanied by a text that talks about what they know and do. When they are photographed in action, they are looking intently at what they are doing, not smiling up at the camera. Nurses on the other hand, rarely are shown focusing intently on their patients, the machines they monitor, or the activities they perform. No, it's always that smile and that glowing gaze straight into the lens of sentimentality.

But is that what nurses look like when they talk to patients, administer and monitor their treatments, help diagnose their problems, and make sure their diseases and treatments don't kill them? Today, the media often rejects nurses as subjects of stories because they perceive nursing to be too touchy-feely. Imagine what a change of image—a few less smiles and a few more serious pictures—would do for the media depiction of nursing.

But the thesis of this collection goes further than a critique of misrepresentation through sentimentalization. Contributors point to a far more insidious problem caused by a sentimentalized caring discourse. When Marie Heartfield worries that the caring discourse may help nurses conceal the very uncaring actions and attitudes they are encouraged to take and adopt, she points to a solution: caring can be used to help nurses fight the kind of economic rationalization that is sweeping health care. When Aranda and Brown warn against disaggregating body work from emotional work, they also point out the power of combining these two activities. And when Tom Keighley alerts us to the dangers of an obsessive focus on health that overshadows the realities of illness, he helps us understand that nurses must mobilize themselves and their societies so that the sick are not scapegoated and are in fact served by those whose role it is to give care when health—even health within illness—is no longer possible.

Finally, a major issue we hope nurses will further debate is the way that the current focus on the feelings-and-relational aspect of nursing work helps to conceal the scientific and (let's say it out loud) medical knowledge and skills nurses master in order to deliver quality care. It might even be called nursing's dirty little secret. And we all know secrets come at a cost. If we tell no one, then no one knows. If we emphasis the hand-holding and special moments, no one will understand the challenge of making patients feel cared for and safe in a terrifying and life-threatening situation. No one gets it that skilled nurses require highly developed interpersonal skills to deliver complex clinical interventions. In fact, the calm and supportive caring nurse is actually controlling his or her emotions so that the patient does not panic and the family can cope with the emergency or devastating diagnosis. This is skilled work at its highest level.

Moreover, when nurses refuse to emphasize their medical knowledge and insight they lose a platform of legitimacy that is crucial to the demand that nurses be acknowledged as full partners of the medical team and in patient care/medical decisions. As we listen to nurses talk about the "medical model," the disease focus of medicine, medicine's lack of holism and so forth, we are struck by the implicit medicine bashing that goes on routinely in nursing. Any doctor listening to the text and/or subtext might realistically conclude that nurses have no interest in diseases, only in the people who have them. If this is the impression nurses—albeit inadvertently— give, is it a surprise that physicians are reluctant to talk to nurses about what they consider to be "medical" issues?

When we were recently talking to the dean of a prestigious U.S. nursing school, she complained that elected officials in her county had just set up a board of clinicians to do long-range planning regarding health issues. Unfortunately, no nurses were asked to serve on the board. The dean approached one of the elected officials on the committee and said, "If you really want to focus on health care, you should have a nurse on the board." We suggested that she might consider revising her pitch: "If you really want to have an effective medical system, how can you consider creating a committee that leaves out what researchers have shown to be the early warning and early intervention system in the delivery of effective medical treatment?" And, then she might add, "If you want to move beyond medical treatment to disease prevention and health promotion, nurses are critical."

Perhaps most disturbing of all is the way nursing scholars continue to talk about nursing's holism as if it were a magical, rather than a learned, set of skills. Meanwhile, on the busy hospital floors and on the rounds of the community nurse, sick people are being cared for by nurses who are in fact very grounded, coolheaded, and scientifically and medically skilled. Nurses are neither social workers nor pastoral care workers—though some of these responsibilities and skills do drift over into the nurse's arena. Nurses are skilled clinicians and yet somehow lack a language to talk about their knowledge or their work.

Perhaps this deficit in nursing language is the result of too much abstract theorizing about a profession that is intensely practical and instrumental. But today more than ever, as the health care system, its workforce, and its service delivery is being reengineered under our feet, nurses can little afford to take their eyes off the game.

One is reminded of a joke, popular among scientists a few years ago. Sherlock Holmes and Dr. Watson were on a case, camped out on the wild moors. In the middle of the night Holmes shakes Watson awake and says, "Watson, look at the stars and tell me what you deduce."

Watson looks up and observes: "I see millions of stars, and I know that about them are millions of planets. Given the vast infinity of space it is clear that there must be a planet in a solar system like ours. I thus deduce there must be life in space."

Holmes turns to Watson and declares: "Watson, you fool! Someone's stolen the tent!"

From the education and preparation of nurses, to the discussion of advanced practice, nurses need to refocus on the tent and its contents—the work of nurses, their knowledge, and their skills. Nurses can do this by reclaiming their scientific and medical knowledge, without apology, without it being considered the sign of an "uncaring" nurse or a wannabe doctor. Nurses need to feel comfortable with talking about the scientific and technical realm in which they practice, as well as talking more effectively about the human interpersonal domain. One does not have to choose between these domains. Instead, we should reject the false polarity set up by much nursing curricula, professional, and even scientific discourse. By rejecting sentimentalization, nursing can start the long overdue process of celebrating what it knows and does. Not only will that make today's nurses willing to stand up for the practice, it will assert the importance of nursing to the care of our citizens. Perhaps most important, it will send the right message that will attract those who would make good nurses. That way we may still have a chance to recruit enough nurses to create a safe and effective health care system in the future.

Notes

1. Moving beyond the Virtue Script in Nursing

1. J. Sochalski, "Nursing Shortage Redux: Turning the Corner on an Enduring Problem," *Health Affairs* 21, no. 5 (2002): 157.

2. C. Czaplinski and D. Diers, "The Effect of Staff Nursing on Length of Stay and Mortality," *Medical Care* 36, no. 12 (1998): 1626–38; L. H. Aiken, S. P. Clark, et al., "Hospital Nurse Staffing and Patient Mortality, Nurse Burnout, and Job Dissatisfaction," *Journal of the American Medical Association* 288, no. 16 (2002): 1987–2041; J. Needleman, P. Buerhaus, et al., "Nurse Staffing Levels and Quality of Care in Hospitals," *New England Journal of Medicine* 346, no. 22 (2002): 1715–22.

3. S. Gordon, B. Buresh, et al., "Who Counts in News Coverage of Health Care?" *Nursing Outlook* 39, no. 5 (1991): 204–8.

4. S. Nelson, *Say Little, Do Much: Nursing, Nuns, and Hospitals in the Nineteenth Century* (Philadelphia: University of Pennsylvania Press, 2001).

5. Ibid., 48.

6. Ibid., 123.

7. S. Reverby, *Ordered to Care: The Dilemma of American Nursing, 1850–1945* (Cambridge: Cambridge University Press, 1996).

8. S. Nelson, "From Salvation to Civic: Service to the Sick in Nursing Discourse," *Social Science and Medicine* 52, no. 9 (2001): 1217–25.

9. C. Rosenberg, *The Cholera Years: The United States in 1832, 1849, and 1866* (Chicago: University of Chicago Press, 1962).

10. M. J. Peterson, *The Medical Profession in Mid-Victorian London* (Berkeley: University of California Press, 1978); R. Porter, *The Greatest Benefit to Mankind* (London: Fontana Press, 1999).

11. (Gull) *The Times* (London) (1880): 9.

12. Peterson, *Medical Profession*, 184–85.

13. Rosenberg, *Cholera Years*, 231.

14. *The Times* (London), Guy's Hospital (December 21, 1886): 8.

15. C. Rosenberg, *The Care of Strangers: The Rise of America's Hospital System* (New York: Basic Books, 1987).

16. B. Abel-Smith, *A History of the Nursing Profession* (London: Heinemann, 1975); A. Bashford, "Frances Gillam Holden and the Children's Hospital Dispute, 1887: Woman's Sphere, Feminism, and Nursing," *Women's History Review* 2, no. 3 (1993): 219–30.

17. Reverby, *Ordered to Care*; J. Moore, *Zeal for Responsibility* (Athens: University of Georgia Press, 1988).

18. Rosenberg, *Care of Strangers*, 218.

19. Abel-Smith, *A History*, 197; S. Forsyth and J. Godden, "Defining Relationships and Limiting Power: Two Leaders of Australian Nursing, 1868–1904," *Nursing Inquiry* 7, no. 1 (2000): 10–19.

20. K. Schultheiss, *Bodies and Souls: Politics and the Professionalization of Nursing in France, 1880–1922* (Cambridge: Harvard University Press, 2001).

21. E. D. Baer, P. D'Antonio, et al., *Enduring Issues in American Nursing* (New York: Springer Publishing, 2001).

22. Fenwick, "Editorial," *Nursing Record and Hospital World* (1901).

23. Rosenberg, *Care of Strangers*, 235.

24. S. Nelson, "From Salvation to Civics: Service to the Sick in Nursing Discourse," *Social Science and Medicine* 52, no. 9 (2001): 1217–25.

25. National Student Nurses Association, *Nursing: The Ultimate Adventure*, video (New York: National Student Nurses Association, 2000).

26. "Ohio Health Celebrates Nursing Excellence Week, May 5–12, 2002" (brochure).

27. *Nursing Profile* (cover copy), October 2001.

28. Honor Society for Nursing, Sigma Theta Tau International, "Nurses for a Healthier Tomorrow," 30-second TV PSA.

29. MUSC Medical Center, *The Many Faces of Nursing* (Charlestown, S.C.: MUSC, 2002).

30. Ibid., 5.

31. "Saint Joseph's Angel of Mercy" (photo), *Toronto Star*, February 9, 2002.

32. W. Taylor, "Angel in Our Midst," *Toronto Star*, February 9, 2002.

33. J. E. Brody, "Premature Births Rise Sharply, Confounding Obstetricians," *New York Times*, April 8, 2003, D5.

34. C. Reeve, *Still Me* (New York: Random House, 1998).

35. Ibid.

36. C. Reeve, *Nothing Is Impossible* (New York: Random House, 2002).

37. Interview by Suzanne Gordon with campaign consultant Laurie Culwell.

38. Johnson & Johnson, "Television Advertising 2002 and Nurse Recruitment," *The Campaign for Nursing's Future*, video (Johnson & Johnson, 2002).

39. Ibid.

40. Johnson & Johnson, "Patient's Perspectives," *The Campaign for Nursing's Future*, video (Johnson & Johnson, 2002).

41. J. H. Packard, "On the Training of Nurses for the Sick," *Boston Medical and Surgical Journal* 95, no. 20 (1876).

42. N. Dickenson-Hazard, "New Harris Poll Is Sobering Wake-up Call for Profession," *Excellence in Clinical Practice* 2 (2002).

2. When Little Things Are Big Things

1. D. B. Weinberg, *Code Green: Money-Driven Hospitals and the Dismantling of Nursing* (Ithaca: Cornell University Press, 2003).

2. S. Gordon, *Life Support: Three Nurses on the Front Lines* (Boston: Back Bay Books, 1997); S. Gordon, *Nursing against the Odds: How Health Care Cost Cutting, Media Stereotypes, and Medical Hubris Undermine Nurses and Patient Care* (Ithaca: Cornell University Press, 2005).

3. M. A. Blegen, C. J. Goode, et al., "Nurse Staffing and Patient Outcomes," *Nursing Research* 47 (1998): 43–50; C. Kovner and P. J. Gergen, "Nurse Staffing Levels and Adverse

Events following Surgery in US Hospitals," *Journal of Nursing Scholarship* 30 (1998): 315–21; L. Aiken, D. M. Sloane, et al., "Organization and Outcomes in Inpatient AIDS Care," *Medical Care* 35 (1999): 948–62.

4. Aiken et al., "Organization and Outcomes."

3. Pride and Prejudice

1. M. C. Belcher, "I'm No Angel," *American Journal of Nursing* 104, no. 7 (2004): 13.

2. S. R. Germain, "Learning the Bones," *American Journal of Nursing* 104, no. 1 (2004): 47.

3. "More Letters: 'Learning the Bones'," *American Journal of Nursing* 104, no. 4 (2004): 70–73.

4. J. Fallows, *Breaking the News: How the Media Undermine American Society* (New York: Vintage Books, 1996).

5. T. Schwarz, "PTSD in Nurses," *American Journal of Nursing* 105, no. 3 (2005): 13.

4. Moral Integrity and Regret in Nursing

1. "Who Will Care for Each of Us? America's Coming Health Care Labor Crisis," in *A Report from the Panel on the Future of Health Care: Labor Force in a Graying Society* (Chicago: University of Illinois, Nursing Institute, 2001).

2. Because the difficulties nurses face in maintaining integrity are exacerbated by the fact that the vast majority of nurses are female, I use the feminine pronoun throughout this chapter. Men make up only 5.4% of the nursing population (U.S. Department of Health and Human Services, *The Registered Nurse Population* [Washington, D.C.: Government Printing Office, 2000], 8).

3. For definitions of integrity, see G. Taylor, "Integrity," *Proceedings of the Aristotelian Society* 55 (1971): 143–59; A. Rorty, "Integrity: Political, Not Psychological," in *Integrity in the Public and Private Domains*, ed. A. Montefiore and D. Vines (London: Routledge, 1982); L. McFall, "Integrity," *Ethics* 98, no. 1 (1987): 5–20: M. Halfon, *Integrity: A Philosophical Inquiry* (Philadelphia: Temple University Press, 1989); B. J. Winslow and G. R. Winslow, "Integrity and Compromise in Nursing Ethics," *Journal of Medicine and Philosophy* 16, no. 3 (1991): 309; C. Calhoun, "Standing for Something," *Journal of Philosophy* 92, no. 6 (1995): 235–60; J. Childress, "Conscience and Conscientious Actions in the Context of MCOs," *Kennedy Institute of Ethics Journal* 7, no. 4 (1997): 403–11.

4. Traits universally incompatible with integrity include hypocrisy, compulsive lying, and cowardly avoidance of difficulty. Such traits by definition involve acting against what one believes to be true or right.

5. Versions of this claim have recently been made by D. Wong, "On Flourishing and Finding One's Identity in a Community," *Midwest Studies in Philosophy* 13 (1988): 324–41; C. Korsgaard, *The Sources of Normativity* (Cambridge: Cambridge University Press, 1996); H. Frankfurt, *The Importance of What We Care About* (Cambridge: Cambridge University Press, 1988); O. Flanagan, *Varieties of Moral Personality: Ethics and Psychological Realism* (Cambridge: Harvard University Press, 1991).

6. For a history of this image of nursing, see B. Melosh, *"The Physician's Hand": Work Culture and Conflict in American Nursing* (Philadelphia: Temple University Press, 1982).

7. See L. Aiken, "Nurses," in *Handbook of Health, Health Care, and the Health Professions* (New York: Free Press, 1983), 407–31; S. Reverby, *Ordered to Care: The Dilemma of American Nursing, 1850–1945* (Cambridge: Cambridge University Press, 1987), 55; J. Wilson-Barnett, "Ethical Dilemmas in Nursing," *Journal of Medical Ethics* 12, no. 3 (1986): 123–26, 135.

8. See http://www.discovernursing.com.

9. L. Curtin, "The Nurse-Patient Relationship: Foundation, Purposes, Responsibilities, and Rights," in *Nursing Ethics: Theories and Pragmatics*, ed. L. Curtin and M. J. Flaherty (Bowie, Md.: Robert J. Brady, 1982).

10. See, for instance, J. H. Penticuff, "Conceptual Issues in Nursing Ethics Research," *Journal of Medicine and Philosophy* 16, no. 3 (1991): 235–58. "What dominates nurses' self-conceptualization in the professional literature is a view of the nurse as giving, caring, advocating for others; always competent, capable, and adequate to the task." There is also a tendency to extend the standard of caring beyond the nurse's actual tasks and to apply it to the nurse herself. As Hilary Graham puts it: "Caring touches simultaneously on who you are and what you do." Quoted by Reverby, *Ordered to Care*, 1.

11. Reverby, *Ordered to Care*, 132.

12. On the unique moral status of the health care professions see R. Gillon, "More on Professional Ethics," *Journal of Medical Ethics* 12, no. 2 (1986): 59–60.

13. For the limitations of thinking of nursing in terms of role, see Penticuff, "Conceptual Issues in Nursing Ethics Research," 243–44.

14. I am limiting myself to the case of hospital nurses since their struggles seem most acute; nurses in private practices and nurse practitioners do not always share these experiences.

15. For discussions of nurses' lack of autonomy in hospital settings, see Penticuff, "Conceptual Issues in Nursing Ethics Research," 244. Again, we might be tempted to say that this power inequality is ubiquitous in employment situations, not unique to nurses. That nursing's plight is unique is argued again by nursing's dealings with life and death and with nurses' especially close identification with their occupation.

16. For a discussion of possible legitimate reasons for this hierarchy, see T. May, "The Nurse under Physician Authority," *Journal of Medical Ethics* 19 (1993): 223–27; P. Nash, "Doctors and Nurses Once More—an Alternative to May," *Journal of Medical Ethics* 21 (1995): 82–83. I should emphasize that this is not the only source of nurses' job dissatisfaction. Another frequently cited problem is the increasing number of patients they are expected to care for in a managed health environment. This too, they claim, inhibits their ability to care for patients as they feel they should. I focus on the physician-nurse relationship because it brings out more clearly the unique nature of the stress nurses experience. Because I am discussing nurses' perception of their powerlessness, I will also not attempt to give the physician's side of the story here.

17. Analyzing nursing as a subordinate position is a central part of Melosh's work; see also A. W. Pike, "*I Don't Know How Ethical I Am": An Investigation into the Practices Nurses Use to Maintain Their Moral Integrity* (Ph.D. diss., Boston University, 2001).

18. For a taxonomy of uses of "care," see J. Blustein, *Care and Commitment: Taking the Personal Point of View* (Oxford: Oxford University Press, 1991).

19. For case studies of this particular dilemma, see C. Mitchell, "Integrity in Interpersonal Relationships," in *Responsibility in Health Care*, ed. G. Agich (Holland: D. Riedel Publishing, 1982); J. Liaschenko and A. J. Davis, "Nurses and Physicians on Nutritional Support: A Comparison," *Journal of Medicine and Philosophy* 16, no. 3 (1991); P. Benner, "Discovering Challenges to Ethical Theory in Experience-Based Narratives of Nurses' Everyday Ethical Comportment," in *Health Care Ethics: Critical Issues*, ed. J. F. Monagle and D. C. Thomasma (Frederick, Md.: Aspen Publishers, 1994).

20. Soma Hewa and Robert W. Hetherington describe this difference as a central component of nursing's struggle: "While the medical profession and health care administrators are attempting to expand the utilization of technological devices in medicine, members of the nursing profession are striving to cope with their humanitarian consequences. Therefore, nurses are trapped between two competing paradigms." S. Hewa and R. W. Hetherington, "Specialists without Spirit: Crisis in the Nursing Profession," *Journal of Medical Ethics* 16 (1990): 179–84.

21. For specific references to loss of integrity in nursing, see Pike, "*I Don't Know How Ethical I Am"*; Mitchell, "Integrity in Interpersonal Relationships"; Winslow and Winslow, "Integrity and Compromise in Nursing Ethics." Penticuff writes that "nursing ethics research that examines how moral integrity is maintained or eroded is significant to understanding

nursing ethical practice because if nurses do not have the will to practice ethically, the entire enterprise of nursing as a helping profession is in jeopardy" ("Conceptual Issues in Nursing Ethics Research," 247).

22. As one nurse put it to me, "If your source of self-esteem is that you are a caring person, but you are not allowed to express that caring, you lose your self-esteem."

23. Pike, "*I Don't Know how Ethical I Am*", 1.

24. For a history of this movement, see Melosh, "*Physician's Hand*", 37–76.

25. A. Bradshaw, "The Virtue of Nursing: The Covenant of Care," *Journal of Medical Ethics* 25 (1999): 477–81.

26. Hewa and Hetherington, "Specialists without Spirit."

27. C. Maslach, *Burnout: The Cost of Caring* (Englewood Cliffs, N.J.: Prentice-Hall, 1982).

28. See, for instance, A. M. Nordhaus-Bike, "Where Have All the RNs Gone?" *Hospitals and Health Networks* 72, no. 8 (1998); M. A. Costello, "Nurses' Work Conditions in the Spotlight: Nursing Counsel Says One Key Is Improving Work Environment," *AHA News* 37, no. 6 (2001); M. Glabman, "Nurses Needed—STAT!" *Trustee* 54, no. 6 (2001).

28. For the argument that bioethics principles cannot transfer directly to nursing ethics, see Penticuff, "Conceptual Issues in Nursing Ethics Research," 235–58; Pike, "*I Don't Know How Ethical I Am*", 108–9; Benner, "Discovering Challenges to Ethical Theory," 402. Liaschenko and Davis argue that "biomedicine developed within the Cartesian framework of separation of mind and body; with this separation, the body became amenable to mechanical explanation, causal laws, and technical intervention. . . . In contrast, the origin of nursing did not arise from an endorsement of such separation and always maintained the centrality of the patient in the restoration of health" ("Nurses and Physicians," 272)

30. Reverby, *Ordered to Care*, 207.

31. Davis and Liaschenko, "Nurses and Physicians," 277; see also Melosh, "*Physician's Hand*", 240.

32. R. B. Marcus, "Moral Dilemmas and Consistency," *Journal of Philosophy* 77, no. 3 (1980): 121–36.

33. Marcus focuses on guilt as the expression of moral distress; following Pike's research on nurses, I will focus on regret. Clearly there are important differences between the two, but I think they are not relevant here.

34. Marcus, "Moral Dilemmas and Consistency," 131.

35. Ibid., 133.

36. Pike, "*I Don't Know How Ethical I Am*", 63–64.

37. Ibid., 175.

38. Ibid., 89.

39. Ibid., 93.

40. Ibid., 3. For further vivid description of nurses' daily struggles, see Suzanne Gordon, *Life Support: Three Nurses on the Front Lines* (Boston: Back Bay Books, 1997).

41. Compare Winslow and Winslow, "Integrity and Compromise in Nursing Ethics," on integrity-preserving compromises, 317.

5. Ethical Expertise and the Problem of the Good Nurse

1. M. Weber, *Politik als Beruf* (Munich: Gesammelte Politische Schriften, 1919); H. H. Gerth and C. W. Mills, *From Max Weber: Essays in Sociology* (New York: Oxford University Press, 1946), 77–128; J. Minson, *The Prince's New Clothes: Why Australians Hate Their Politicians* (Sydney: University of New South Wales Press, 2002).

2. Weber, *Politik als Beruf*, 77.

3. Ibid., 78

4. Ibid., 77

5. Benner et al., *Expertise in Nursing Practice: Caring, Clinical Judgment, and Ethics* (New York: Springer, 1996); P. Benner, "A Dialogue between Virtue Ethics and Care Ethics," *Theo-*

retical Medicine 18 (1997): 47–61; P. Benner, "The Roles of Embodied Emotion and Lifeworld in Nursing Practice," *Nursing Philosophy* 1, no. 1 (2000): 5–19.

6. P. Benner, *From Novice to Expert* (Menlo Park, Calif.: Addison-Wesley, 1984).

7. C. Gilligan, *In a Different Voice: Psychological Theory and Women's Development* (Cambridge: Harvard University Press, 1982).

8. P. Benner, *From Novice to Expert.*

9. S. Nelson and M. McGillion, "Expertise of Performance? Calling into Question Narrative Use in Nursing," *Journal of Advanced Nursing* 47, no. 6 (2004): 631–38.

10. Benner et al., *Expertise in Nursing Practice*, 350.

11. Study of Nursing Education, Carnegie Foundation for the Advancement of Teaching, http://www.carnegiefoundation.org/aboutus/staff/benner.htm.

12. Benner, *From Novice to Expert*, 31, 32.

13. Ibid.

14. Benner, et al., *Expertise in Nursing Practice*, 355. See Nelson and McGillion, "Expertise or Performance," for a full discussion of the methodological issues in Benner's narrative approach.

15. Benner et al., *Expertise in Nursing Practice*, 378, 356.

16. Ibid., 255.

17. A. MacIntyre, *After Virtue: A Study in Moral Theory* (London: Duckworth Press, 1981).

18. J. Tully, ed., *Philosophy in an Age of Pluralism: The Philosophy of Charles Taylor in Question* (Cambridge: Cambridge University Press, 1994).

19. N. Smith, *Charles Taylor* (London: Polity Press, 2002).

20. P. Benner, "The Role of Articulation in Understanding Practice and Experience as Sources of Knowledge in Clinical Nursing," in J. Tully, ed., *Philosophy in an Age of Pluralism*, 136–58.

21. C. Taylor, "Charles Taylor Replies," in *Philosophy in an Age of Pluralism*, ed. J. Tully, 213–57.

22. Benner, "Roles of Embodied Emotion," 12.

23. Ibid., 11.

24. Benner et al., *Expertise in Nursing Practice*, 326.

25. MacIntyre, *After Virtue*, 181.

26. Benner et al., *Expertise in Nursing Practice*, 6.

27. Dreyfus et al., "Implications of the Phenomenology of Expertise."

28. Benner et al., *Expertise in Nursing Practice*, 168.

29. Ibid., 47.

30. Dreyfus et al., "Implications of the Phenomenology of Expertise."

31. Benner et al., *Expertise in Nursing Practice*, 168.

32. Ibid., 152.

33. Ibid., 154.

34. Ibid., 12.

35. Ibid., 162.

36. Benner, "A Dialogue," 54.

37. C. Taylor, *Sources of the Self: The Making of Modern Identity* (Cambridge: Cambridge University Press, 1989), 362.

38. Benner, in J. Tully, ed., *Philosophy in an Age of Pluralism*, 143.

39. Benner et al., *Expertise in Nursing Practice*, 331.

40. Ibid., 267, 266.

41. J. Rubin, "Impediments to the Development of Clinical Nursing Knowledge and Ethical Judgment in Critical Care Nursing," in Benner et al., eds., *Expertise in Nursing Practice.*

42. Ibid., 187.

43. Ibid., 182.

44. Benner et al., *Expertise in Nursing Practice*, 118–22.

45. Ibid., 161.

46. S. Callahan, "The Role of Emotion in Ethical Decision Making," *Hastings Centre Report* 18, no. 3 (1988): 9–14.

47. Rubin, "Impediments to the Development of Clinical Nursing," 190, 189.

48. Ibid., 189.

49. Ibid.

50. Nelson and McGillion, "Expertise or Performance?"

51. S. Nelson and M. E. Purkis, "Mandatory Reflection: The Canadian Reconstitution of the Competent Nurse," *Nursing Inquiry* 11, no. 4 (2004): 247–57.

52. Rubin, "Impediments to the Development of Clinical Nursing."

53. Benner et al., *Expertise in Nursing Practice*, 275.

54. Ibid.

55. Ibid., 154.

56. MacIntyre, *After Virtue*.

57. Benner et al., *Expertise in Nursing Practice*, 332–35.

58. Ibid., 348.

59. R. Rudge, "Reflections on Benner: A Critical Perspective," *Contemporary Nurse: A Journal for the Australian Nursing Profession* 1 (1992): 84–88; S. M. Padgett, "Benner and Her Critics: Promoting Scholarly Dialogue," *Scholarly Inquiry for Nursing Practice: An International Journal* 14, no. 3 (2000): 249–65.

60. L. H. Aiken, S. P. Clarke, et al., "Education Levels of Hospital Nurses and Surgical Patient Mortality," *Journal of the American Medical Association* 290 (2003): 1617–23; S. P. Clarke and L. H. Aiken, "Registered Nurse Staffing and Patient and Nurse Outcomes in Hospitals: A Commentary," *Policy, Politics, and Nursing Practice* 4, no. 2 (2003): 104–11.

61. S. James, "The Good-Enough Citizen," in *Beyond Equality and Difference: Citizenship, Feminist Politics, and Female Subjectivity*, ed. G. Bock and S. James (London: Routledge, 1992).

62. Dreyfus et al., "Implications of the Phenomenology of Expertise," 268.

63. D. F. Chambliss, *Beyond Caring: Hospitals, Nurses, and the Social Organization of Ethics* (Chicago: University of Chicago Press, 1996).

64. Ibid., 184.

65. Gilligan, *In a Different Voice*.

66. S. Gordon and S. Nelson, "An End to Angels," *American Journal of Nursing* 105, no. 5 (2005): 62–69.

67. Ibid.

6. From Sickness to Health

1. World Health Assembly, Declaration of Alma-Ata (1978), doc. no. WHA30.43, Geneva, World Health Organization.

2. B. Harmer and V. Henderson, *Textbook of the Principles and Practice of Nursing* (New York: Macmillan, 1939).

3. V. Henderson, *A Definition of Nursing* (Geneva: International Council of Nurses, 1960).

4. ICN, "The ICN Definition of Nursing" (Geneva: International Council of Nurses, 2002), pamphlet.

5. Australian Nursing Council, *Code of Professional Conduct for Nurses in Australia* (Canberra: ANC, 2004).

6. Canadian Nurses Association, *Code of Ethics for Registered Nurses* (Ottawa: CNA, 2002).

7. Royal College of Nursing, *Defining Nursing* (London: RCN, 2003).

8. Sigma Theta Tau, *The Society's Vision and Mission* (Indianapolis: Sigma Theta Tau International Honor Society of Nursing, 2004).

9. J. Palmer, "On Patient Obligations," *Health Service Journal* (2004): 19.

10. A. V. Campbell, *Moderated Love: A Theology of Professional Care* (London: SPCK, 1984).

7. The New Cartesianism

1. S. Gordon, *Life Support: Three Nurses on the Front Lines* (Boston: Back Bay Books, 1997).

2. P. Benner and J. Wrubel, *The Primacy of Caring: Stress and Coping in Health and Illness* (Menlo Park, Calif.: Addison-Wesley, 1989).

3. Ibid., 33.

4. Ibid., 34.

5. Ibid., 41.

6. Ibid., 42.

7. Ibid., 43, 49.

8. J. Baker-Miller, *Toward a New Psychology of Women* (Boston: Beacon Press, 1976); M. Field Belenky et al., *Women's Ways of Knowing: The Development of Self, Voice, and Mind* (New York: Basic Books, 1986); C. Gilligan, *In a Different Voice: Psychological Theory and Women's Development* (Cambridge: Harvard University Press, 1982).

9. M. Sandelowski, *Devices and Desires: Gender, Technology, and American Nursing* (Chapel Hill: University of North Carolina Press, 2000), 180.

10. B. D'Angio, sample exemplar from the Circle of Excellence Award applications (Aliso Viejo, Calif.: American Association of Critical Care Nurses), brochure.

11. S. Gordon, *Nursing against the Odds: How Health Care Cost Cutting, Media Stereotypes, and Medical Hubris Undermine Nurses and Patient Care* (Ithaca: Cornell University Press, 2005).

12. F. E. Katz, "Nurses," in *The Semi-Professions and Their Organization: Teachers, Nurses, Social Workers*, ed. A. Etzioni (New York: Free Press, 1969).

13. Sandelowski, *Devices and Desires*, 11.

14. Ibid., 180.

15. Johnson & Johnson, "Patient Perspectives," *The Campaign for Nursing's Future*, video (Johnson & Johnson, 2002).

16. "Quiet Power," *Nursing Standard* (2005), DVD by Nick Shipley, produced by Nursing Standard.

17. Gordon, *Life Support*.

8. Nurses Must Be Clever to Care

1. S. K. Aranda and J. M. Parker, "Nursing Practices in Malignant Wound Care," (manuscript); S. K. Aranda, "A Critical Praxis Study of Nursing-Patient Friendship," La Trobe University, Melbourne, 1998.

2. F. Nightingale, *Notes on Nursing: What It Is and What It Is Not* (London: Harrison and Sons, 1859; repr. New York: Churchill Livingstone, 1980).

3. R. A. Dingwell, A. Rafferty, et al., *An Introduction to the Social History of Nursing* (London: Routledge, 1988).

4. D. Armstrong, "The Fabrication of Nurse-Patient Relationships," *Social Science and Medicine* 17, no. 8 (1983): 457–60.

5. D. E. Orem, "The Self-Care Deficit Theory of Nursing: A General Theory," in *Family Health—A Theoretical Approach to Nursing Care*, ed. I. Clements and F. Roberts (New York: Wiley Medical, 1983).

R. R. Parse, *Man-Living-Health—A Theory of Nursing* (New York: John Wiley and Sons, 1981).

6. J. Watson, *Nursing: The Philosophy and Science of Caring* (Boston: Little, Brown, 1979).

7. Armstrong, "Fabrication of Nurse-Patient Relationships."

8. Ibid.

9. I. Menzies, "A Case-Study in the Functioning of Social Systems as a Defense against Anxiety: A Report on a Study of the Nursing Service of a General Hospital," *Human Relations* 13, no. 2 (1960): 95–121.

10. C. A. Tanner, P. Benner, et al., "The Phenomenology of Knowing the Patient," *Journal of Nursing Scholarship* 25, no. 4 (1993): 273–80.

11. P. Benner and J. Wrubel, *The Primacy of Caring: Stress and Coping in Health and Illness* (Menlo Park, Calif.: Addison-Wesley, 1989).

12. C. P. Tresolini, *Health Professions, Education, and Relationship-Centered Care* (San Francisco: Pew Health Professions Commission, 1994).

13. A. Pearson, "Trends in Clinical Nursing," in *Primary Nursing: Nursing in the Burford and Oxford Nursing Development Units,* ed. A. Pearson (London: Croom Helm, 1988).

14. R. McMahon, "Therapeutic Nursing: Theory, Issues and Practice," in *Nursing as Therapy,* ed. R. McMahon and A. Pearson (London: Chapman and Hall, 1991); K. Kadner, "Therapeutic Intimacy in Nursing," *Journal of Advanced Nursing* 19 (1994): 215–18; S. Ersser, "Nursing Beds and Nursing Therapy," in Pearson, ed., *Primary Nursing*; S. Ersser, "A Search for the Therapeutic Dimensions of Nurse-Patient Interaction," in McMahon and Pearson, eds., *Nursing as Therapy.*

15. J. Parker and S. Aranda, "The Decaying Body and Palliative Care in Nursing." Unpublished research study. University of Melbourne School of Nursing, 2003.

16. J. Lawler, *Behind the Screens: Nursing, Somology, and the Problem of the Body* (Melbourne: Churchill Livingstone, 1991).

17. All names are psuedonyms except for the research nurse Brown.

18. D. Shapiro, *Mom's Marijuana: Insights about Living* (New York: Harmony Books, 2000), 88.

19. Ibid., 89.

20. Ibid.

21. Aranda and Parker, "Nursing Practices in Malignant Wound Care."

22. Aranda, "A Critical Praxis Study," 175.

23. A. F. Street, *Inside Nursing: A Critical Ethnography of Clinical Nursing Practice* (Albany: State University of New York Press, 1992).

24. Aranda, "Critical Praxis Study."

25. N. James and D. Field, "The Routinization of Hospice: Charisma and Bureaucratization," *Social Science and Medicine* 34, no. 12 (1992): 1363–75.

26. L. A. Copp, "The Spectrum of Suffering," *American Journal of Nursing* 74 (1974): 491–95; A. J. Davis, "Compassion, Suffering, Morality: Ethical Dilemmas in Caring," *Nursing, Law, and Ethics* 2 (1981): 1–2, 6.

27. D. W. Kissane, "Death and the Australian Family," in *Death and Dying in Australia,* ed. A. Kellehear (Melbourne: Oxford University Press, 2000).

28. Aranda, "Critical Praxis Study," 138, 169.

9. "You Don't Want to Stay Here"

1. M. Heartfield, "Governing Recovery: A Discourse Analysis of Hospital Length of Stay" (Ph.D. diss., University of Melbourne, 2002).

2. D. Lupton, "Discourse Analysis: A New Methodology for Understanding the Ideologies of Health and Illness," *Australian Journal of Public Health* 16 (1992): 145–50.

3. E. D. Baer, C. Fagan, et al., *Abandonment of the Patient: The Impact of Profit-Driven Health Care on the Public* (New York: Springer, 1996); D. Allen, *The Changing Shape of Nursing Practice: The Role of Nurses in the Hospital Division of Labour* (London: Routledge, 2001); A. Clarke and R. Rosen, "Length of Stay," *European Journal of Public Health* 11, no. 2 (2001): 166–70.

4. E. von Dietze and A. Orb, "Compassionate Care: A Moral Dimension of Nursing," *Nursing Inquiry* 7, no. 3 (2000): 166–74; G. Andrews, "Towards a More Place-Sensitive Nursing Research: An Invitation to Medical and Health Geography," *Nursing Inquiry* 9, no. 4 (2002): 221–38.

5. J. Latimer, *The Conduct of Care* (Oxford: Blackwell Science, 2000); Allen, *Changing Shape of Nursing Practice,* 2001; R. Dingwell and D. Allen, "The Implications of Healthcare Reforms for the Profession of Nursing," *Nursing Inquiry* 8, no. 2 (2001): 64–77.

6. S. Gordon, *Life Support: Three Nurses on the Front Lines* (Boston: Back Bay Books, 1997).

7. J. Liaschenko, "The Shift from the Closed to the Open Body: Ramifications for Nurs-

ing Testimony," in *Philosophical Issues in Nursing*, ed. S. D. Edwards (London: Macmillan, 1998).

8. Allen, *Changing Shape of Nursing Practice*, 177.

9. C. M. Fagin, *When Care Becomes a Burden* (New York: Milbank Memorial Fund, 2001).

10. J. Needleman, P. Buerhaus, et al., *Nurse Staffing and Patient Outcomes in Hospitals* (Boston: Health Resources Services Administration, 2001); L. H. Aiken, S. P. Clarke, et al., "Hospital Staffing, Organisation, and Quality of Care: Cross-National Findings," *International Journal of Quality in Health Care* 14, no. 1 (2002): 5–13.

11. National Centre for Classification in Health, *Strategic Plan 2000–2005* (Brisbane, 2000).

12. Ibid.

13. M. Foucault, "Governmentality," in *The Foucault Effect: Studies in Governmentality*, ed. G. Burchell, C. Gordon, and P. Miller (Chicago: University of Chicago Press, 1991).

14. P. O'Malley, "Risk and Responsibility," in *Foucault and Political Reason: Liberalism, Neo-Liberalism, and Rationalities of Government*, ed. N. Rose (Chicago: University of Chicago Press, 1996).

15. Latimer, *Conduct of Care*; M. Heartfield, "Regulating Hospital Use: Length of Stay, Beds and Whiteboards," *Nursing Inquiry* 12, no. 1 (2005): 21–26.

16. N. J. Fox, "Anaesthetists, the Discourse on Patient Fitness and the Organisation of Surgery," *Sociology of Health and Illness* 16, no. 1 (1994): 1–18.

17. J. Latimer, "Writing Patients, Writing Nursing: The Social Construction of Nursing Assessment of Elderly Patients in an Acute Medical Unit" (Ph.D. diss., University of Edinburgh, 1993).

18. C. Wiener, "Holding American Hospitals Accountable: Rhetoric and Reality," *Nursing Inquiry* 11, no. 2 (2004): 82–90.

19. T. Osborne, "Of Health and Statecraft," in *Foucault, Health, and Medicine*, ed. A. Peterson and R. Bunton (London: Routledge, 1997).

20. N. Rose, *Powers of Freedom: Reframing Political Thought* (Cambridge: Cambridge University Press, 1999).

21. Suzanne Gordon, personal communication, 2003.

22. Clarke and Rosen, "Length of Stay."

23. P. Johnstone and G. Zolese, "Length of Hospitalisation for People with Severe Mental Illness," *Cochrane Database of Systematic Reviews*, 2 (1999); P. Langhorne, *Services for Reducing Duration of Hospital Care for Acute Stroke Patients* (Oxford: Cochrane Library, 2000); J. Parkes and S. Sheppard, *Discharge Planning from Hospital to Home* (Oxford: Cochrane Library, 2000).

24. Clarke and Rosen, "Length of Stay."

25. M. E. Purkis, "Managing Home Nursing Care: Visibility, Accountability and Exclusion," *Nursing Inquiry* 8, no. 3 (2001): 141–50.

26. C. Cordery, "Doing More with Less: Nursing and the Politics of Economic Rationalism in the 1990s," in *Issues in Nursing*, vol. 4, ed. R. Pratt (Melbourne: Churchill Livingstone, 1995).

27. Langhorne, *Services for Reducing Duration of Hospital Care*; Parkes and Sheppard, *Discharge Planning*; Purkis, "Managing Home Nursing Care."

28. F. Nightingale, *Notes on Nursing* (London: Scuteri Press, 1992).

29. S. Nelson, *A Genealogy of Care of the Sick* (Southsea Hants, U.K.: Nursing Praxis Press, 2000), 1.

30. World Health Organization, *Declaration of Alma-Ata* (Geneva: WHO, 1978); World Health Organization, *The Ottawa Charter for Health Promotion* (Geneva: WHO, 1986).

31. A. Wass, *Promoting Health: The Primary Health Care Approach* (Marrickville, New South Wales: Harcourt W. B. Saunders, 2000); F. Baume, "Community Health Research," in *Health for All: The South Australian Experience*, ed. F. Baume (Adelaide: South Australian Community Health Research Unit and Wakefield Press, 1995).

10. Research on Nurse Staffing and Its Outcomes

1. G. S. Wunderlich, F. A. Sloan, et al., *Nursing Staff in Hospitals and Nursing Homes: Is It Adequate?* (Washington, D.C.: National Academy Press, 1996).

2. S. P. Clarke and L. H. Aiken, "Registered Nurse Staffing and Patient and Nurse Outcomes in Hospitals: A Commentary," *Policy, Politics, and Nursing Practice* 4, no. 2 (2003): 104–11.

3. S. P. Clarke, "Balancing Staffing and Safety," *Nursing Management* 34, no. 6 (2003): 44–48.

4. M. Baernholdt and N. M. Lang, "Why an ICNP? Links among Quality, Information, and Policy," *International Nursing Review* 50 (2003): 73–78.

5. Clarke, "Balancing Staffing and Safety."

6. L. I. Iezzoni, *Risk Adjustment for Measuring Healthcare Outcomes* (Chicago: Health Administration Press, 1997).

7. Clarke, "Balancing Staffing and Safety."

8. L. H. Aiken, E. T. Lake, et al., "Design of an Outcomes Study of the Organization of Hospital AIDS Care," *Research in the Sociology of Health Care* 14 (1997): 3–26; L. H. Aiken and D. M. Sloane, "Effects of Organizational Innovations in AIDS Care on Burnout among Urban Hospital Nurses," *Work and Occupations* 24 (1997): 453–77.

9. B. A. Mark,. A. J. Salyer, et al., "What Explains Nurses' Perceptions of Staffing Adequacy?" *Journal of Nursing Administration* 32, no. 5 (2002): 234–42.

10. http://www.nursingquality.org.

11. See, for instance, D. Doran, *Nursing Sensitive Outcomes: The State of the Science* (Sudbury, Mass.: Jones and Bartlett, 2003).

12. Baernholdt and Lang, "Why an ICNP?"

13. P. Benner, "Relational Ethics of Comfort, Touch, and Solace—Endangered Arts?" *American Journal of Critical Care* 13, no. 4 (2004): 346–49.

14. C. Kovner, C. Jones, et al., "Nurse Staffing and Postsurgical Adverse Events: An Analysis of Administrative Data from a Sample of U.S. Hospitals, 1990–1996," *Health Services Research* 37, no. 3 (2002): 611–29.

15. J. Needleman, P. Buerhaus, et al., "Nurse Staffing Levels and Quality of Care in Hospitals," *New England Journal of Medicine* 346, no. 22 (2002): 1715–22.

16. S. P. Clarke, "The Policy Implications of Staffing-Outcomes Research," *Journal of Nursing Administration* 35, no. 1 (2005): 17–19.

17. G. E. P. Box, "Robustness Is the Strategy of Scientific Model Building," in *Robustness in Statistics*, ed. R. L. Launer and G. N. Wilkinson (New York: Academic Press, 1979).

18. P. I. Good and J. W. Hardin, *Common Errors in Statistics (and How to Avoid Them)* (Hoboken, N.J.: Wiley-Interscience, 2003).

19. Clarke, "Policy Implications."

20. A. Zuger, "Dissatisfaction with Medical Practice," *New England Journal of Medicine* 350, no. 1 (2004): 69–75.

21. Baernholdt and Lang, "Why an ICNP?"

22. L. H. Aiken and S. P. Clarke, et al., "Hospital Nurse Staffing and Patient Mortality, Nurse Burnout, and Job Dissatisfaction," *Journal of the American Medical Association* 288, no. 16 (2002): 1987–93.

23. J. Buchan, "A Certain Ratio? Minimum Staffing Ratios in Nursing" (London: Royal College of Nursing, April 2004), http://www.rcn.org.uk/downloads/news/minimum-staffing-ratios-april29.doc.

24. Clarke, "Balancing Staffing and Safety"; Clarke, "Policy Implications."

25. Joint Commission on Accreditation of Healthcare Organizations, *Front Line of Defense: The Role of Nurses in Preventing Sentinel Events* (Oakbrook Terrace, Ill.: Joint Commission on Accreditation of Healthcare Organizations, 2001).

26. L. A. Callaghan, D. W. Cartwright, et al., "Infant to Staff Ratios and Risk of Mortality

in Very Low Birthweight Infants," *Archive of Diseases in Childhood: Fetal and Neonatal Edition* 88 (2003): F94–F97.

Conclusion

1. Julie Sochalski, "Nursing Shortage Redux: Turning the Corner on an Enduring Problem," *Health Affairs* 21 (2002): 159, 161.

Contributors

SANCHIA ARANDA, RN, PhD, is Professor/Director of Cancer Nursing Research at the Peter MacCallum Centre, and Head of the University of Melbourne School of Nursing. Since 1979 she has worked in cancer and palliative care in practice, research, and teaching. She has more than forty publications, including refereed journal articles, book chapters, and conference proceedings, and has been joint editor of two significant Australian palliative care texts. She is co-consulting editor of the *International Journal of Palliative Nursing* and President of the International Society of Nurses in Cancer Care.

ROSIE BROWN is an experienced nursing clinician and a Master of Nursing by Research student at the University of Melbourne School of Nursing.

SEAN CLARKE, RN, PhD, CRNP, is Assistant Professor of Nursing at the University of Pennsylvania School of Nursing. He is a nursing workforce researcher and Associate Director of Penn's Center for Health Outcomes and Policy Research. He is a Senior Fellow of the Leonard Davis Institute of Health Economics at Penn. He serves on the National Nursing Advisory Council of the Joint Commission on Accreditation of Healthcare Organization's Sentinel Event Review and is an adjunct faculty member at the Université de Montréal, the largest university school of nursing in the French-speaking world.

SUZANNE GORDON is an awarding-winning journalist and author. She is coeditor of the Culture and Politics of Health Care Work series for Cornell University Press. She is author of over three hundred articles that have appeared in such publications as the *New York Times* and the *Boston Globe*. She is the author or editor of ten books, including *Nursing against the Odds: How Health Care Cost Cutting, Media Stereotypes, and Medical Hubris Undermine Nurses and Patient Care* and *Life Support: Three Nurses on the Front Lines*.

MARIE HEARTFIELD, RN, PhD, is the Program Director of Research Degrees in the University of South Australia's School of Nursing and Midwifery. Her research interests include the contribution of nursing to health care and issues of practice, policy, and regulation. She is reviewing the Competency Standards for Registered Nurses on behalf of the Australian Nursing and Midwifery Council.

TOM KEIGHLEY has practiced and taught general, psychiatric, and community nursing. He has served as an adviser in national policy formulation at the Royal College of Nursing and on management boards at the district and regional level. He founded the Institute of Nursing at the University of Leeds and has served as Director of International Development in its School of Healthcare Studies. He has served as the UK representative of the Practising Profession of Nursing on the Advisory Committee for the Training of Nurses in Brussels and advises British government departments and the European Commission on related issues. He has been the editor of *Nursing Management*. In 2001 he was awarded the Gran Cruz de ASO FAME for services to health care in Columbia. In 2003, he was ordained as a minister in the Anglican Church. In 2004, he was awarded the Fellowship of the Royal College of Nursing.

DIANA J. MASON, RN, PhD, FAAN, is the editor in chief of the *American Journal of Nursing*. She is the coproducer and moderator of *Healthstyles*, a weekly radio program on health, health care, and health policy.

LYDIA L. MOLAND is Assistant Professor of Philosophy at Babson College in Wellesley, Massachusetts. She has held fellowships at the American Academy in Berlin and at the Liguria Study Center in Bogliasco, Italy. She writes on Hegel and concepts of moral integrity.

SIOBAN NELSON, PhD, is Dean of the Faculty of Nursing at the University of Toronto. Her clinical background is acute medical-surgical nursing; her principal research interests are in the history of nursing, health policy, and professional issues. She is coeditor of the Culture and Politics of Health Care Work series for Cornell University Press and editor of the international journal *Nursing Inquiry*. She is the author of a history of religious nursing and hospital foundation, *Say Little, Do Much: Nurses, Nuns, and Hospitals in the Nineteenth Century*, and *A Genealogy of Care of the Sick*.

DANA BETH WEINBERG, PhD, is Assistant Professor of Sociology at Queens College, the City University of New York. She is author of *Code Green: Money-Driven Hospitals and the Dismantling of Nursing* in the Culture and Politics of Health Care Work series of Cornell University Press.

Index

advanced practice nurses, 2, 6, 13, 123
aging nursing workforce, 13, 38, 99
aging population, 13, 181
AIDS care, 169–70
AIDS/HIV epidemic, 98
Aiken, Linda, 10
American Association of Critical Care Nurses (AACCN), 114
American Journal of Nursing, 8, 44–46
American Nurses Association, 20, 21, 46, 96, 170
angels, nurses as: and critical debate, 44, 48; and virtue script, 18, 20, 21, 22, 25, 26, 54, 186
Aquinas, Thomas, Saint, 73, 76, 84
Aranda, Sanchia, 9–10, 136, 187, 188
Aristotle, 73, 74, 76, 77, 83–84, 85
Australia, 2, 19, 71, 127, 144
Australian Nursing Council, 90–91
authenticity, 5, 6

Benner, Patricia: and Cartesianism, 107, 108; and definition of expertise, 8, 70–71, 83; and disposition towards the good, 69, 73, 74, 76, 79, 82; and emotional work, 7, 79, 80; and intuition, 78, 82, 84; and moral agency of nurse, 77, 78; and nursing as moral practice, 75–76, 86, 87; and practice narratives, 72–73, 77, 79, 81, 83; and seven moral skills, 74, 83; and Taylor, 73–74; and voice, 85

Beth Israel Hospital, Boston, 7–8, 28, 30–33, 40–42, 104, 119
Box, George, 174
Bradshaw, Ann, 60
Brazil, 2
Britain, 19, 27–28, 97, 99, 100, 101
British Columbia Nurses Union, 28, 187
Buresh, Bernice, 187
burnout, 31, 40, 41, 48, 60, 170

Callaghan, L. A., 183
Callahan, S., 80
Canada, 13, 19, 71, 81
Canadian Nurses Association, 21, 91, 96
caring: as art of self, 4; cost of, 11; definitions of, 3, 5, 6, 51, 56, 57, 59, 65–66, 67, 123
caring discourse: and Cartesian mind/body divide, 106–8, 117, 118; as dogma, 11; and emotional work, 56–57, 104, 108–9; and families, 110, 114; and models of nursing care, 8; and nurse-patient relationship, 7, 10, 114, 124, 125–26; and nursing practice, 3–4, 56–57, 125, 185, 186; and patient outcomes, 84; and professionalization of nursing, 60, 125; and self-understanding, 53, 55, 59, 60, 61, 67–68, 194n10; and technical/medical expertise, 5, 57, 188; and virtue script, 7
caring for sick/vulnerable: as health care system's core mission, 9; and health dis-

caring for sick/vulnerable (*cont.*)
course, 90–93, 95, 96–97, 100; and nursing
profession, 88, 89, 90, 101–2; and nursing
shortages, 11; and public understanding,
100; and stigmatizing of the sick, 98–99,
100, 102, 103
Cartesian mind/body divide: and caring
discourse, 106–8, 117, 118; and devaluing
of technical/medical expertise, 109–12,
116, 121; and holism, 9, 106; implications
of, 118–21; and invisibility of nursing
care, 112–13, 121; and nursing education,
106, 117; and nursing practice narratives,
109–10, 113, 114–15, 118; rebellion against,
107–9; and technical/medical expertise,
106, 113
Chadwick, Edwin, 18
Chambliss, Daniel, 85–86
chronic illness, 13, 154
Clarke, Sean, 10–11
Clifford, Joyce, 31
Code Green (Weinberg), 7–8, 30
cost-cutting measures: and caring discourse, 3, 120–21; and ethics, 83; and
health discourse, 98, 100; and hospital
length of stay, 10, 145; and nursing care,
1–2, 32, 141–42; and nursing practice, 9,
123, 185; and virtue script, 28
credible voice: and ethical expertise, 85; and
public understanding, 3; silencing of, 45;
and virtue script, 26
critical debate: and images of nurses, 8, 44–
46, 48–49; in society, 46–47

Danish Nurses Organisation, 96
Declaration of Alma-Ata of 1978, 9, 88, 93,
94, 95–96, 101, 158
Descartes, René, 107
Devices and Desires (Sandelowski), 112–13
Dreyfus, Hubert, 80, 85

Electronic Medical Record, 170, 172
emotional work: and authenticity, 5; and
caring discourse, 56–57, 104, 108–9; and
Cartesian mind/body divide, 106, 107;
expertise involved in, 7, 79, 80, 82, 120;
focus on, 4, 114, 123; and holism, 9; importance of, 11, 56; and moral integrity,
57; and nursing organizations, 3; physical
care contrasted with, 129–35; and self-
understanding, 57, 60; and staffing ratios,
161; and therapeutic use of self, 48
ethics: codes of, 91; and cost-cutting mea-

sures, 83; and expertise, 8, 69, 74, 75–76,
77; Gallup poll on, 49; individual ethics,
75; medical ethics compared with nursing
ethics, 61, 195n29; and nursing organizations, 3; and nursing practice, 87; and
plurality of ethical conduct, 69–70; and
repertoire of ethical capacities, 82. *See also*
moral integrity
expertise: in caring for the sick, 102; definition of, 70–71, 74, 83; and ethics, 8, 69, 74,
75–76, 77; experienced but not expert, 79–
81, 82, 85, 86, 87; and failure to achieve
mastery, 84–85, 86; measures of, 87; narratives of, 72–73, 77, 79, 81, 83, 85, 87; and
recognition of the good, 76–79, 84, 87. *See
also* knowledge work; technical/medical
expertise

families: and blaming individual nurses, 4;
and caring discourse, 110, 114; and ethical
expertise, 79; and nurse-patient relationship, 35; nurses' conflicts with, 50; nursing as service to, 90, 102
Federation of Nurses of Quebec, 21
feedback loop, and virtue script, 7, 15, 21,
22, 23, 25
feminism, 61, 70, 108
Foucault, Michel, 109, 148
France, 19
From Silence to Voice (Buresh and Gordon),
187

Gallup polls, 25–26, 49
Gilligan, Carol, 70, 86, 108
Gordon, Suzanne, 9, 26, 28–29, 34, 86, 146,
154, 186, 187
guilt, 4, 61–62

Harris polls, 25–26
health care policymakers: and caring discourse, 3; and hospital length of stay, 156,
157; and nursing research on staffing, 163,
165; and nursing shortage, 13
health care systems: and caring discourse,
5–6; and health discourse, 9, 98–99; and
market models, 123; and models of nursing care, 13–14; nurses' conflicts with, 50,
57, 194n20; and nurses' ethics, 84, 85, 86,
87; and nurses' regret, 51, 62, 66; nursing's role in, 7, 11, 118; restructuring of, 4,
9, 10, 30; and socioeconomic status, 98
health discourse: changes in, 93–99; effect
of, 8–9; and hospital length of stay, 158;

and nursing organizations, 9, 89, 90–93, 96, 99; and nursing practice, 98, 100–101; and stigmatizing of the sick, 98–99, 100, 102, 103, 188
Heartfield, Marie, 10, 188
Heidegger, Martin, 107
Henderson, Virginia, 89, 90
holism and holistic rhetoric: and caring discourse, 122, 125; and Cartesian mind/body divide, 9, 106; domination of, 6; and health discourse, 95, 98; and hospital length of stay, 154, 155, 156; and knowledge work, 9, 116; and nurse-physician relationship, 189; and nursing practice, 9, 112, 115, 119; and virtue script, 26, 28
Hong Kong, 2
hospice care, 138–39
hospital beds, 147, 148, 150, 155, 156, 159
hospital length of stay: decline in rate of, 146–47; and nurse-patient relationship, 143–44, 148–49, 151–52, 155, 156; and nursing care, 155–57; and nursing practice, 149, 156, 157–58, 159; and preadmission clinics, 150–53; and prerecovered patients, 149–50, 153–55; and recasting surgical event, 148–50; as rigid standard, 159; and time as resource, 145–46
hospitals: and caring for the sick, 100; history of, 146; and images of nurses, 188; integrity of nursing services in, 7; and market models, 123, 150; and Nightingale, 18; and nurse retention, 31; and nurses' conflicts with management, 50; and nursing profession, 15–16, 17; and preadmission clinics, 147, 150–53; restructuring of, 30–31, 42, 145

identity, and moral integrity, 52, 54, 55
images of nurses: and complexity of care concepts, 67; and critical debate, 8, 44–46, 48–49; historical formation of, 14; and recruitment, 187, 188; and virtue script, 15, 20–21, 23–24, 116
industrialization, 15
integrity. See moral integrity
International Council of Nurses (ICN), 89–90
Ireland, 2

James, Susan, 84–85
Johnson & Johnson Campaign for Nursing's Future, 7, 23–24, 27–29, 53, 118, 187

Joint Commission on Accreditation of Healthcare Organizations, 170, 180

Keighley, Tom, 8–9, 188
knowledge work: decomplexifying of, 3; and holism, 9, 116; and nurse-patient relationship, 34–37, 130, 131; and nurse staffing, 1; and nursing education, 2; and nursing practice, 8, 54, 104, 162; and nursing research on staffing, 177, 182–83; and physical care, 123, 128, 130, 131–32, 140; and virtue script, 7, 14, 16–17, 19, 20, 21, 25–27, 29; and women's roles, 15–16. See also technical/medical expertise

legitimacy: critical debate on, 8; and emotional work, 130; and nurses' status, 89; and nursing profession, 18–19, 26; and patient outcomes, 84; public legitimacy, 3; and recruitment campaigns, 14; and virtue script, 20, 26
Liaschenko, Joan, 146, 195n28
Life Support (Gordon), 104, 105, 120
Lippincott, Jay, 46
Locke, John, 107

MacIntyre, Alisdair, 73, 75–76, 78, 82
Malone, Beverly, 20, 186
Maslach, C., 60
Mason, Diana, 8
Massachusetts Nurses Association, 21
media representations: and images of nurses, 188; and knowledge work, 26; and virtue script, 7, 15, 22
medical profession, history of, 17, 55, 93–94
Medical University of South Carolina, 21–22, 25, 26
men: and nurse retention, 86; in nursing profession, 13; and virtue scripts, 27; and women's role in nursing profession, 15
Menzies, Isabel, 126
Moland, Lydia, 8
Mom's Marijuana (Shapiro), 132
moral integrity: and contradictions in work, 8, 50; and moral dilemmas, 8, 61–62, 63, 64, 65, 66, 67, 85; and moral distress, 59, 60, 61, 62, 65, 66, 68; and nursing practice, 53, 54, 56, 57, 58–59, 61, 157–58, 160, 195n21; and regret, 50–51, 59–67, 68; and self-understanding, 51, 52–59, 63, 66, 67; traits incompatible with, 193n4. See also ethics
Morley, Barry, 121

National Database of Nursing Quality Indicators, 170
National Health Service (Britain), 97
National Student Nurses Association, 20
Needleman, Jack, 171
Nelson, Sioban, 8, 116
New Zealand, 2
Nightingale, Florence: and caring for the sick, 98, 103; and ideal of doing no harm, 157; and nurse-led management, 9; and nurse-physician relationship, 17, 124; and professionalization of nursing, 76; and reform of nursing, 18, 185; uniform of, 16; and virtue script, 53
Notes on Nursing (Nightingale), 124
nurse leaders, 6, 9, 10, 13
nurse managers: and caring rhetoric, 5, 34; and hospital beds, 147, 148; and Nightingale system, 9; and nursing research on staffing, 179, 180; and nursing workforce restructuring, 83, 130–31; and palliative care, 127–31; and patient care, 100, 123
nurse-patient relationship: and advocacy, 51, 56–59, 63–66, 78, 85, 146; and caring discourse, 7, 10, 114, 124, 125–26; and Cartesian mind/body divide, 106, 107, 108, 110–11, 118–19; conflict in, 4, 50; and economic rationalization in health care, 10, 27; and ethical expertise, 79; and hospital length of stay, 143–44, 148–49, 151–52, 155, 156; and interplay between types of care, 135–40; and job satisfaction, 38–39, 40, 41, 42; and knowledge work, 34–37, 130, 131; meaning of, 6, 9, 35–36, 43; and model of nursing care, 31–32; and moral integrity, 57, 63; and nursing workforce restructuring, 33–35, 38, 42; and physical care, 119, 131–35, 139–41, 142; and sentimentalization of nursing care, 3; and therapeutic use of self, 48, 188–89; and trustworthiness of nurses, 119–20; and virtue script, 23, 24, 26
nurse-physician relationship: and Cartesian mind/body divide, 106, 108; conflict in, 50, 55, 57, 58, 59, 63; history of, 17–18, 19, 55, 59, 124; and holism, 189; and moral integrity, 57, 58, 62–65, 67; and nurses' advocacy for patient, 57, 58, 64–65; and nurses' technical/medical expertise, 117–18; and nursing care, 35, 55–56; and nursing profession, 88, 125; and power relations, 55–56, 194nn15, 16; and professionalization of nursing, 60; and virtue script, 21–23, 25, 26

nurse practitioners, 6, 60, 115
nurse retention: and conflict in workplace, 50; and knowledge work, 29; and men, 86; rates of, 13, 28; and restructuring, 31; and sentimentalization of nursing care, 186
Nurses for a Healthier Tomorrow campaign, 20
nurse staffing: and knowledge work, 1; and regulation of nursing, 3. *See also* nursing research on staffing; nursing workforce restructuring; staffing ratios
Nurses Week campaigns, 20, 21–22, 24–25
Nursing Against the Odds (Gordon), 116
nursing care: and cost-cutting measures, 1–2, 32, 141–42; and hospital length of stay, 155–57; invisibility of, 112–13, 121, 187, 188, 189; models of, 8, 13–14, 28, 31–32; nursing research on staffing, 170–72, 176–78; and patient risk, 14, 104; public understanding of, 105; skilled work inherent in, 126–29, 135, 141, 142; and virtue script, 23. *See also* patient care; physical care; sentimentalization of nursing care
nursing education: Benner's influence on, 71; and Cartesian mind/body divide, 106, 117; and critical debate, 47; history of, 17; and knowledge work, 2; and nursing research on staffing, 178, 181; and patient care, 99; and technical/medical expertise, 114
nursing organizations: and excellence awards, 114–15; and health discourse, 9, 89, 90–93, 96, 99; and images of nurses, 187; and nursing care, 105; and nursing shortage, 13; virtue script and, 20–21, 25
nursing practice: autonomy of, 85; and caring discourse, 3–4, 56–57, 125, 185, 186; challenges of, 7; concrete realities shaping, 4; and cost-cutting measures, 9, 123, 185; and effects of nursing workforce restructuring, 30, 33–34, 38, 42; as ethical form of conduct, 76–77; and ethics, 87; expertise defined in, 70–71, 74, 83; financial resources for, 4, 11; and health discourse, 98, 100–101; and holism, 9, 112, 115, 119; and hospital length of stay, 149, 156, 157–58, 159; idea of the good in, 69, 73–75; and knowledge work, 8, 54, 104, 162; and moral integrity, 53, 54, 56, 57, 58–59, 61, 157–58, 160, 195n21; as moral practice, 75–76, 78, 87; narratives of, 72–73, 77, 79, 81, 83, 85, 109–10, 113, 114–15, 118; and

nurses' regret, 51, 62–64; and nursing research on staffing, 163, 180, 181–82; and patterns of care, 96; public understanding of, 67, 122–23; and rationalist science, 78, 80, 82; and role of nurse, 50; and therapeutic use of self, 48–49; and virtue script, 14, 55, 186

nursing process, 96

nursing profession: as caring, 1; and caring for sick/vulnerable, 88, 89, 90, 101–2; contested space of, 17–18; emergence of, 15–17; goals of, 66; and health discourse, 97–100, 101; hierarchy of goals for, 95; internal cohesion of, 5; and legitimacy, 18–19, 26; and nursing research on staffing, 162–63, 174–81, 183; philosophical issues of, 7, 8, 86; self-definition of, 7, 89, 90–93, 96, 125, 130, 177; and technical/medical expertise, 11, 60, 116, 125; and women's roles, 13, 14, 15–17

nursing research: and hospital length of stay, 155; and nursing care, 32; and nursing practice, 71, 89; and palliative care, 126–29; and patient outcomes, 84; and practice narratives, 72–73, 81; and public university funding, of 2–3; rating of, 2–3

nursing research on staffing: and contributions of human services work, 175–79; dangers in narrow reading of, 179–81; directions of, 162, 181–84; limitations of, 10–11; and measurement techniques, 163–64, 172; nature of, 172–74; nursing care, 170–72, 176–78; and nursing profession, 162–63, 174–81, 183; and patient outcomes, 166–70, 172, 173, 179; and process of care, 170–72; and public understanding, 27, 161–62, 178; as reflection of clinical reality, 163–74; and staffing ratios, 161, 164–66, 172, 173, 179–80, 183

nursing shortages: and aging workforce, 13; and caring discourse, 6; and caring for sick/vulnerable, 11; global scale of, 13; and health discourse, 103; and hospital length of stay, 144; and nursing education, 2; and nursing research on staffing, 174, 181; and nursing workforce restructuring, 41; and recruitment, 14, 27–28, 53; and staffing ratios, 13, 161; and virtue script, 23–24

nursing specializations, 147

nursing workforce restructuring: and deskilled nursing work, 2, 124, 180; effects on nursing practice, 30, 33–34, 38, 42; effects on palliative care, 9, 123, 127, 129, 130–31, 141–42; effects on patient outcomes, 146; and patient risk, 4, 34, 38; and replacing higher skilled workers with less skilled workers, 4, 99, 123; and self-blame, 40

Orem, Dorothea, 125
Ottawa Charter, 158

palliative care: and effects of nursing workforce restructuring, 9, 123, 127, 129, 130–31, 141–42; and nurse-patient relationship, 120, 135–40; skilled work inherent in, 126–29, 137–38

Parker, Judith, 126

Parse, Rosemary, 125

patient care: and caring discourse, 4–5; and coordinators/leaders of care, 6, 9, 10; and expertise, 71; fragmentation of, 123, 124, 131, 135, 188; and hospital length of stay, 144; and nurse managers, 100, 123; nurses' centrality to, 14, 25, 32, 40; and nursing education, 99; and nursing research on staffing, 165, 166–70; and staffing ratios, 161; standards of, 86–87

patient confidentiality, 141

patient mortality: and nurse staffing, 10; and nursing research on staffing, 168–69, 170, 178

patient outcomes: and caring discourse, 84; effects of nursing workforce restructuring, 146; and hospital length of stay, 155; and nursing research on staffing, 166–70, 172, 173, 179; and staffing ratios, 146, 161

patient risk: and critical debate, 47; and hospital length of stay, 155; and nurse-patient relationship, 37, 39; and nursing care, 14, 104; and nursing workforce restructuring, 4, 34, 38; and physical care, 140; and staffing ratios, 10, 41, 51, 161–62, 179, 182

patient self-management: and health discourse, 9; and hospital length of stay, 147, 148, 150, 155, 156, 159; and nurse-patient relationship, 10; resources for, 153, 154, 157

philanthropic movements, 15

physical care: and caring discourse, 125–26; devaluing of, 4, 99, 108–9, 110, 111–12, 116–17, 121, 122, 132, 135; and interplay between types of care, 135–40; and nurse-patient relationship, 119, 131–35, 139–41,

physical care (*cont.*)
142; and nursing workforce restructuring, 124; and palliative care, 123, 126–29; and patient management, 10; and personal space, 102; and staffing ratios, 161; and technical/medical expertise, 113; visibility of, 187
Polara polls, 25–26
political environment: and caring discourse, 3–4; and ethics, 69–70; and knowledge work, 26; and nurse-patient relationships, 43; and nursing profession, 17; and nursing shortage, 13; and public understanding, 3
power relations: and caring discourse, 56; and ethical expertise, 85; and nurse-patient relationship, 136; and nurse-physician relationship, 55–56, 194nn15, 16; and nurses' ethical conflicts, 50–51, 65; and oppressed group behavior, 46, 47–48; and political environment, 70; and virtue script, 21, 25
primary nursing, 32
public health, 93, 95
public understanding: and credible voice, 3; and health discourse, 100, 101; of nurses' scientific knowledge and clinical skill, 14, 118; of nursing care, 105; of nursing practice, 67, 122–23; and nursing research on staffing, 27, 161–62, 178; and virtue script, 15, 20, 27, 28
Purkis, Mary Ellen, 81

Quebec Order of Nurses, 21

recruitment: and images of nurses, 187, 188; and knowledge work, 29, 190; and nursing shortage, 14, 27–28, 53; and sentimentalization of nursing care, 185–86, 188; and virtue script, 7, 14, 15, 19–21, 23–24, 27
reductionism, 107, 109
Reeve, Christopher, 23
registered nurses, 6, 11, 89
regret, and moral integrity, 50–51, 59–67, 68
regulation of nursing, 1, 3, 40
religious nurses, 15, 16, 18, 19
Reverby, Susan, 61
Robb, Isabel Hampton, 19
Rosenberg, Charles, 18, 19
Royal College of Nursing (RCN), 92, 96, 99, 122

salaries, 13, 29, 60
Sandelowski, Margarete, 112–13, 117
Scholasticism, 76
secondary post-traumatic stress, 48
self-blame, 4, 39, 40, 42
self-care deficit model, 125
self-understanding: and caring discourse, 53, 55, 59, 60, 61, 67–68, 194n10; and emotional work, 57, 60; formation of, 53; and health discourse, 98; and identification with profession, 54, 55, 194n15; and moral integrity, 51, 52–59, 63, 66, 67; and patient advocacy, 58; and professionalization of nursing, 60–61; and virtue script, 53, 54
sentimentalization of nursing care: and narratives, 114–15; and nurse-patient relationship, 3; and nurses' blame, 4; and ranking of authenticity, 5; and recruitment, 185–86, 188; rejection of, 190; and virtue script, 7, 21, 26, 27, 28, 116
Shapiro, Dan, 132–33
Sigma Theta Tau International, 20, 92–93
Sochalski, Julie, 186
socioeconomic status: and health discourse, 98–99; and nursing profession, 15, 16
staffing ratios: and hospital length of stay, 156; and moral integrity, 194n16; and nursing research on staffing, 161, 164–66, 172, 173, 179–80, 183; and nursing shortage, 13, 161; and patient outcomes, 146, 161; and patient risk, 10, 41, 51, 161–62, 179, 182; and physical care, 161
Street, Annette, 136
Study of Nursing Education, 71
Swiss Nurses Association, 186, 187
Switzerland, 2
systemic issues, and ethics, 8

Taylor, Charles, 73–74, 78, 79
technical/medical expertise: and caring discourse, 5, 57, 188; and caring for the sick, 102; and Cartesian mind/body divide, 106, 113; devaluing of, 109–12, 116, 121; and holism, 9, 115; and interplay between types of care, 135–40; and invisibility of nursing care, 112–13, 121, 187, 188, 189; as knowledge work, 123; and nurse-patient relationship, 119, 137–38; and nursing as moral practice, 87; and nursing care, 104–5; and nursing profession, 11, 60, 116, 125; reclaiming of, 190; and self-

understanding, 60, 67; and virtue script, 22. *See also* knowledge work

trustworthiness of nurses: and caring discourse, 116; and nurse-patient relationship, 119–20; surveys of, 1, 3, 49, 86, 177; and virtue script, 25, 26

unions: and health discourse, 100; and nursing shortage, 13; and nursing workforce restructuring, 41–42; and professionalism, 42; and staffing ratios, 41
United Kingdom, 2
United States, 13, 19, 27–28, 71, 96, 178

virtue script: and caring discourse, 7; and critical debate, 44; and ethics, 76, 86; and feedback loop, 7, 15, 21, 22, 23, 25; historical formation of, 14, 18–19, 27, 55; and images of nurses, 15, 20–21, 23–24, 116; and

knowledge work, 7, 14, 16–17, 19, 20, 21, 25–27, 29; and nursing practice, 14, 55, 186; and recruitment campaigns, 7, 14, 15, 19–21, 23–24, 27; and self-understanding, 53, 54; and trivializing of complex skills, 11–12
vocational students, 2

Watson, Jean, 125
Weber, Max, 69–70, 87
Weinberg, Dana Beth, 7–8, 28, 121
women's roles: and nursing profession, 13, 14, 15–17; and virtue script, 14
working conditions: and ethics, 83; and nursing shortage, 13; and part-time work, 39–40; and professionalization of nursing, 60; and recruitment, 29; and self-blame, 40
World Health Assembly, 88, 93, 96
World Health Organization, 96